Richard Hath

PANIC ATTACKS
and ANXIETY
HOW TO BEAT THEM

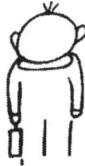

www.astara-publications.com

The author of this book does not dispense medical advice or
prescribe the use of any technique as a form of treatment for
physical or medical problems without the advice of a physician,
either directly or indirectly. The intent of the author is only to
offer information of a general nature to help you in your quest
for physical fitness and good health. In the event you use any of
the information in this book for yourself, the author assumes no
responsibility for your actions.

1st edition Shaking Hands with the Devil 2006

2nd revision Conquering Panic Attacks & Anxiety 2010

3rd revision Panic Attacks & Anxiety - How to beat them 2014

Cover design by BespokeBookCovers.com

ISBN: 978-1-291-65733-3

Praise for Panic Attacks and Anxiety
How to Beat Them

'Wow! What a great book and not written by another doctor who studied the subject but has never experienced it. I actually found a book that describes exactly how I am feeling and can relate to everything in it. Written from the heart and from someone who has experienced it firsthand and helped himself. Written like he is actually talking and supporting all the way through. All the self help is really easy to follow so I feel hopeful that if I follow the course I will conquer my anxiety which has made me like a prisoner in my mind for years. Thank you and well done. A real inspiration!'

Miss Limited Edition

'This book is packed with information that many a reader searching for answers to their condition may not previously have come across and is so easy to understand I found it a joy to read and am already recommending it a lot.'

Anita Childs

'There is a very human feel to the book and I do believe books written about panic attacks are best written by those who have suffered. This is a self help book with a difference. I found it helpful and thought provoking.'

Mrs S.J. Charge

'This book is deep thinking but straight from the heart and I have thoroughly enjoyed reading it. It is nice to know I am not alone, but the author does not feel sorry for himself, and neither am I going to. I am going to try some of the remedies recommended. This is an author I would certainly like to meet.'

Mrs A. Stowers

This book is dedicated to all those suffering with anxiety and panic attacks, and to reassure them, they will get through this.

I wrote this book to make a difference to people's lives.

CONTENTS

A Word from the Author

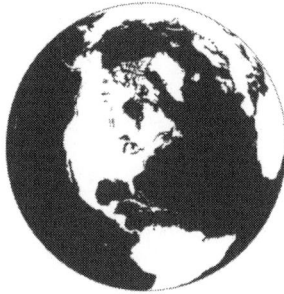

An ever changing world

Since writing the first edition of this book the world has changed beyond recognition. If stress and anxiety was an issue back in 2005, now we see it becoming more of a problem, and the ever increasing sales of the book prove this. The cost of living has risen considerably, yet wages aren't sufficient, and in many cases, unemployment is now the norm only compounding the problem further.

In a world where fuel costs are outweighing food prices, we have a dilemma. People are unable to get to work, or, when they do, there is very little left for the bills and feeding the family. The result? Stress and panic is inevitable. Suicide can also be an option for the desperate. But not a solution.

Credit card bills rise. Loans with APR of twelve hundred percent all offer a quick fix over something that will burst again, and then you come to realise, what you thought had given you some breathing space, has actually only added to the pressure.

You stare in disbelief at your costs, you dread certain days of the month when the next bill hits the mat, because you will have to try and rack your brains in finding a way to pay. Stress stress and more stress. But that's not all, relationships are breaking down. Arguments are becoming more frequent, and all you talk or row about is money and how your life hasn't turned out quite as you had dreamed. And perhaps later you split, and then the anxiety becomes worse than ever, stopping you from working. You feel awful, sick of life and wonder what's in store. You fear you are dying and repeatedly visit the doctors or the hospital only to find out you're fit and well. But you question this; you find it impossible to understand why you feel so bad, and you strongly convince yourself there is in fact something physically wrong.

Eventually, throughout all the trauma this condition brings, you wonder if there is anything you can do about it. Anything to get you back to normal, the person you were before.

And that's the turning point. The point where you take matters into your own hands and take the necessary changes which will lead to your recovery.

Because everybody in their lives will experience the horror that anxiety brings, it just depends on many factors, and how long and to what degree they will suffer this. You may be thinking nobody understands how I feel, I am dying here. But take heart in this, by working through this book, which has evolved through my own experiences of dealing with this dreadful disorder, you will come through this. You will realise that your body is only reacting to a high influx of adrenaline, and the downright, scary, debilitating symptoms are a result of this. And the more these symptoms happen, your body gets used to being in a high state of alert, and when this occurs, it becomes habitual. Your body doesn't feel like it belongs to you anymore, it seemingly reacts to every given danger in a frightening way, and this only compounds your fears further. The vicious circle has begun.

Your mind is the nerve centre, the way your thoughts have become over the day's months and years, contribute to the symptoms you are experiencing. Which is why at the end of the day it will be up to you to beat this. It won't come in a pill bottle, and the doctor won't be able to help with this part, you have to dig down and really want this. No matter how tired and scared you are feeling right now, you must muster up some courage and see this thing through, otherwise it will only become such a big part of you, it will get more and more difficult to eradicate.

People, in way I mean the non suffers, will do their best to help, and you will need the assistance and support of those around you, but still deep down, it will be up to you to combat this.

And that's where this book is designed to assist you. An aid to help you through panic and anxiety as quickly as possible, so you can get on with your life once again. Because nobody wants to feel the clutches this debilitating condition brings. It can be a long tough road, I have fought bouts of this for most of my life, but you do come to realise, although it is horrible, you can get a reign on this.

You see, you are a good person, you have just come over-sensitised to the outside world and you are picking up triggers that would normally mean nothing to a non sufferer, but to you, it feels like death is knocking on your door. Except it isn't death, it's just your body working like it was designed to, but at the moment you don't need it to be so finely tuned. Your overly worked nervous system needs a rest, it needs time to heal, which is why it can take time.

So be gentle with the process, look after yourself, and don't beat yourself up if those intrusive thoughts are driving you crazy. Every day you chip away at this, gradually the feelings will not come with such regularity, and when you finally feel safer in your own body, your path to recovery will be back on track.

But for now, let's work on you, let's get you better.

So remember,

'This is day one of the rest of your life'

Richard Hathaway 2014

- Section One -

Gaining a new Strength

- 1 -

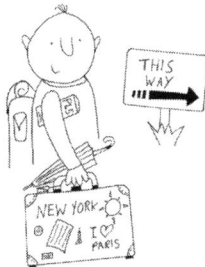

A New Beginning

A quick start into your new healing programme

If you were to ask me today what I'd gained from panic attacks, I'd look at you and smile. Not because I find it a funny question, but because I have come to understand myself better through my mission to search for an answer. And that's what it's all about, it's about finding you, the you who you were born to be, and moving away from the person you are right now. It's an opportunity of a lifetime. It's better than winning the lottery, it's better than anything monetary or material wise. It's about finding the real you and having the inner calm and self confidence that says, 'you know what, I can do anything.'

But where does panic come from? How is it you feel so bad without seemingly doing anything? – Good questions, but firstly let me say this statement. *'Whatever the negative thought, it has an equal reaction to the body.'*

Which makes sense. Fear makes your body sweat, it shakes, you feel as though you want to run, you feel sick. That maybe from just thinking a place is scary, or the people within.

But nevertheless, it happens because deep down in your subconscious you allow it to happen. If you went into the situation saying to yourself it holds no fear for you, you'll go in and the feelings will not materialize. – Panic is just this negative response that has gone on overdrive. For one reason or another, the body has become over sensitive, and every little thing makes you feel awful. And yes, that can be something simple like just coping with day to day living.

Our brains, not dissimilar to a computer's hard drive, becomes written with negative thinking, which needs to be cleared and replaced with positive. By doing this, the body responds in a harmonic manner and panic leaves without trace. Game over for panic, new beginnings for you.

It sounds simple, and in a sense it is, but don't become disheartened if progress is slower than you hope. It has taken a while to get to the stage you are in today, and so likewise, it can take time when returning to a place of well being.

So how did it happen? How did panic come about when you thought on the whole life was being handled okay?

That's easy, how we as a planet live, that's how.

Have you ever stood and wondered where we as a human race are heading as an entirety? What's going to happen if things continue as they are, and will we all end up in one giant ball of stress wondering where life is taking us?

Because if you look at it, that's where many of us are heading. The world has become one long rush, and our bodies are saying enough's enough, I can't cope with this anymore. And who can blame them. The pressure to have the right house, the car, the acceptable kind of job is enormous. Forget who the person is, forget if they are a genuine soul; only think of them in material terms.

It becomes a battle to have the best of everything, and to do this, nearly every hour is spent working. The remainder leaves us cramming in the shopping, picking the kids up from school, and dropping them off at clubs or friends. – There is no quality time. A period just to relax and be.

Panic doesn't come about solely because you were beaten up in year eight during a tough term at school. It's there through an accumulation of things like a hectic lifestyle, how you've been treated in the past, and how you are expected to behave by others. Which is why anger, along with frustration, is such a big player when we look at this. Politeness mixed with fear suppresses what needs to be said or done. And instead of releasing anger, it becomes pent up inside creating more anger. But eventually that anger needs to come out in one shape or form. Panic is just a release valve for this.

Some thoughts that contribute towards anxiety attacks:

O **I can't cope.**

O **Where am I going with my life?**

O **Why is it I never get anywhere and other people do?**

O **Why do people constantly put me down?**

O **Why do I always get the problems?**

O **I'm useless; I don't deserve to be here.**

O **Everything I do fails, why bother.**

O **I feel scared, I don't want all this.**

Leading to thinking along with the attacks themselves:

O Fear of dying.

O Fear of losing control.

O Fear of losing mind.

O Fear there is something physically wrong.

O Fear when the next attack might strike.

O Fear if the next attack will be worse.

O Fear of the pain.

O Fear of choking to death.

O Fear of what's happening.

O Fear of what others might think of you.

This kind of thinking panics the mind which turns the body into one of the most natural responses we have today, the fight or flight response. Something we are all born with, but when it happens, it can be confusing and very frightening. – (More on this later).

But at least we know the panic attacks are nothing to worry about now, it's a natural response to a perceived danger. Yet this can be reversed. The response can be de-sensitized so you can live the life you always wanted, and not be living in fear wondering when the next attack will strike.

First steps towards recovery

It's never easy starting upon something new, and when it comes to a recovery process of any sorts, it's often seen as a long drawn out affair where the end result isn't always satisfactory. But luckily, this isn't true where panic attacks are concerned, because you can beat them and lead a normal life again. – That may sound a long way off, or in your mind, perhaps impossible. But negative thinking like this can hold you back, while locking you firmly in that very same place you feel you're stuck in right now.

So instead of thinking, 'I can't do this,' think, 'I can do this.' And although this looks a small step from the outside, in fact this is an immensely powerful tool and one you will learn more about later in the book. - The power of positive self talk.

But firstly, let me introduce something that will help, yet be completely safe with any medication you may be presently on. Natural remedies have proved very beneficial for many people, including myself, and I wholly recommend them in your recovery programme.

Bach flower Rescue Remedy

Rescue Remedy is very good for panic attack sufferers because of its ability to get things back into perspective, giving you a stronger base to work from. You know from your own experience, it's always easier to deal with a problem when you are feeling calm and in a positive state of mind. Rescue Remedy helps with this.

The five flower extracts are:

Rock Rose   The remedy for rescuing from terror – Panic.

Clematis   Feelings of vacant and inattentiveness.

Prefers to be alone.

Avoids difficulties by withdrawing.

Cherry Plum Fear of mind giving way.

Impatiens   For impatience, irritability and nervousness.

Star of Bethlehem   Counteracts severe shock.

Rescue Remedy is the first port of call in any emergency. It can be taken in the mouth, on the lips, or rubbed on any pressure point throughout the body.

'*Take every ten minutes in severe cases, otherwise every hour to calm the panic feelings.*'

Getting hold of some Rescue Remedy

I realise some of you might be confined to your homes, either through deep fear, or a physical disability, and are unable to get some for yourself. Luckily you can do one of the following.

○Ask a family member or friend to get you some. Rescue Remedy is widely available from most chemists, health food shops, and supermarkets.

○Look up in the yellow pages under homeopathic doctors and see if there is a home delivery service.

○Order over the internet. There are many online shops.

Visit: www.creaturecomforters.co.uk

○Ask your G.P. if he knows of any Bach remedy practitioners in your area.

Basic affirmations

Affirmations have long been recognised as a very good way of changing problematic thinking into positive ones. The two below are very simple, yet don't let that fool you into thinking they are a waste of time. They are highly effective in the early stages of your healing, and should be said as many times as you can during the coming months. Make them your new healing mantra.

Say: 'I am willing to change', &, 'I am getting stronger.'

And although this might seem rather futile at first glance, it's actually kick starting your brain to run a path of positive. Which means, instead of the negative thoughts bouncing around up there, what you're doing is a bit of positive psychology. You're giving yourself permission to change, which is different from someone else telling you.

It's like anything. We trust the ideas we come up with, we want control. But if someone forces an idea, you back away and say, 'I'll think about it, mull it over.' You love to come up with the solutions yourself because its independence, and I guess at the end of the day it has to be your own personal gut feeling, otherwise the devotion or belief shall never be there. If it fails under someone else's idea you'll give up easily and pass blame. 'Oh well, I knew it wouldn't work.' Your idea however, and you'll fight to make it work. That's belief with determination.

By saying *'I am willing to change'*, &, *'I am getting stronger'*, it might hurt a bit, tears can flow under emotion while a fear of the future creeps in. But nevertheless, the act of giving yourself permission to move forward is a big leap. Before, you've been tied up in who you've become over the years, unable to break free. Now authorization has been laid on the table, it's like receiving all your Christmas presents at once. *'You can change. Really, it's okay to be you.'*

We'll discuss more of this later. But for now, take the Rescue Remedy and try and relax because you are in good hands.

Moving things further

Once you've been using the Rescue Remedy and felt the benefits, it's going to come as no surprise that taking the flower remedies a stage further would be advantageous. Many healers use Bach remedies as an addition to their main healing, and there are practitioners out there who deal solely with them. Either way, you'll want to hunt one out in the next week or two and make an appointment. I would have never bounced back without this method, and would still be wandering the wilderness in some kind of haunted daze waiting for the next attack to strike. By using remedies on a regular basis, they have helped me deal with the problems that caused the attacks in the first place, bringing issues to the forefront of my mind so I could release them fully and move forward.

And now if I look back, yes I've suffered, yes it's been a horrendous ride. And yes, there where times when I curled up on the floor in severe pain wishing the world to swallow me. But it got better through trying a host of different avenues. And if I'd failed to do that, I wouldn't be in a position to help you, which is now my priority.

So if you're screaming a kind of scared madness from inside, looking for answers, and feel lower than ever before, at least there's something you can turn to during any moment of the day and get relief. Techniques proven to work so you don't have to feel mad, or think your life is ending in tormenting pain. There are ways which I'm all too happy to show you.

What can I expect by taking Rescue Remedy?

You'll feel stronger within. I can't water this all down, but the truth is, you might have to sort through some pretty tough stuff from your life, 'Real Moments' that caused the 'Big Problems,' and still do for one reason or another. Just don't fear the process ahead. It may cause all kinds of emotional turmoil, but as you work through, you'll begin to notice certain things won't affect you as much, which is empowering in itself.

How about if I'm taking Beta Blocker's (anti-depressants), or thinking about taking them?

Concerning beta blocker/anti-depressants. All the therapies and techniques in this book work fine when taking beta blockers. If you feel you need them and they are helping, great. But remember, if you should want to come off them, please consult your doctor first.

And if you are thinking about taking them but wonder what they do, read further. Beta blockers do what they say. Block. They block the messages the brain is giving the body to react in a panic situation. Faster heart beat, tensing of the muscles etc. Many people feel that they help keep the anxiety down, so if you do decide to take them, keep to the regime the doctor gives you. You can still have healing and do everything I mention in the book, don't worry, eventually your doctor will gradually wean you off. But you have to remember, it's vital not to stop suddenly when dealing with beta blockers or any other anti-anxiety drugs.

In the past, I have helped people taking them and not. It doesn't seem to slow the process, it just means you have to be careful not to build up a dependency on them. (Fearing panic will return if you stop taking them). The aim of this process is to beat anxiety as naturally as you can, but if you can't cope without anxiety drugs, then so be it, use whatever tools you need to overcome this.

At the end of the day, it's a personal preference thing, and something best talked over with those nearest you and your doctor.

What else can I do?

Seize some early nights for starters - Get back some of the energy you've lost through nervous exhaustion. Like the sleepless nights and continual stress which all take their toll on the body's system.

Eat well - Nourish the body and take good care of yourself. You deserve this pampering. And remember the big world out there will survive pretty damn fine if you have a break once in a while. Cities won't fall, order won't crumble, and civilisation for sure won't end.

Stimulants - However tempting they may be, keep off any stimulants such as tea, coffee and chocolate. In fact anything which contains caffeine/refined sugar is a no no. They will only make the symptoms far worse and in some cases even trigger an attack. Try drinking plenty of water to cleanse the system, *(2L is the recommended daily dosage)* although avoid sparkling. Gas makes an already sensitive stomach very painful, accompanied by terrific heart burn fuelling the possible thought you're going to die. So please, for sanity's sake, keep to the still water.

'As a tip, just add a few drops of Rescue Remedy to a glass of water and sip throughout the day. You drink naturally anyway, and this diminishes the chance of forgetting your remedy.'

And if you happen to be a heavy caffeine junky, don't go cold turkey. You'll need to wean yourself back off by gradually reducing your intake, otherwise the effects of sudden withdrawal can be dramatic in the least. The same goes for smokers.

'To recap, it's a good idea to stay away from: Alcohol, smoking, coffee, tea, chocolate, sweets, gassy drinks, and

most cold medicines. In fact anything that contains a stimulant such as caffeine. Food or drink which can increase the chance of wind is also best avoided.'

Top tips: *'Add a few drops of Rescue Remedy to a glass or bottle of water and sip throughout the day.'*

'Also, find somebody who can encourage you through this.'

Now sit back, breathe deeply, and rest in the knowledge you're now in the best possible hands. I'm now committed to helping you, and while there are no time limitations to full recovery, the right track has been found and soon enough you'll be feeling better.

As for the moment, remember to use the remedy with the affirmation. Both are highly important so don't relax on either. Please take the utmost care, looking after yourself is very much the key.

Summary

Tick

Box

☐ Get hold of some Rescue Remedy.

☐ Have a consultation with a Bach flower therapist.

☐ Take time out & have some early nights.

☐ Stay away from stimulants (e.g. caffeine).

☐ Eat well and at regular times.

☐ For the moment, continue with any medication you are on.

☐Beta blockers/anti-depressants. It's okay to take them if you feel you need them. But don't come off them without consulting your doctor first.

☐Don't be afraid to talk about your feelings with a trusted friend.

☐Remember, 'YOU ARE SAFE.'

- 2 -

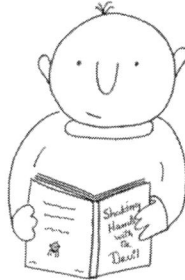

How to use this Book

Although there are no strict rules on how to approach your new healing programme, I'd strongly advise you to read this book from cover to cover, and then go back re-reading and trying the exercises. By doing this, your overall understanding of the condition will rise dramatically; which in turn throws water over the raging flames currently burning within. Or put another way, our knowledge of what's happening to us when an attack occurs dampens the power it has over us. Because panic fuels further panic, leading to more panic. Take the fear away, and things are starting to feel different already.

I'm not trying to simplify what you're feeling right now, I'm merely sign posting the way so you can gain the strength needed to defend yourself against attacks. This helps you understand the areas of your life which are the source of the problem.

There may be one problem, or a whole nucleus of problems, but with strength the human spirit will conquer all. - It's rather like Star Wars, good against evil. Light against dark. Light always beats dark no matter how deep the hole might be. You shall do the same. Yet it can take time. Years of past negative thoughts have become fixed tight upon the brain, etched there for you to gently scrub piece by piece until completely removed.

You'll have to don a pair of theoretical marigolds and get stuck in with the similar theoretical detergent. But however tough it might be, moving forward is better than not moving at all.

'Remember, the future now beckons, the past is just history.'

But I just can't concentrate, what else can I do?

If you're suffering badly right now and reading a book is the last thing on your mind, then rest assured I can still help. I understand you don't want to read, the discomfort is too great and words on the page make little sense, which is why I have put together a *'Survival Kit'* (see chapter 26). This kit was the first thing I knew I had to do for you, because when pain comes to the point of madness, where do you turn?

The therapist is otherwise engaged. The doctor has a waiting list so long you can't see him, and as for the hypnotherapist, he's out of the country. However, don't despair, in your hands you have something more valuable than all the money in this world of ours, a saviour, a Survival Kit.

It's a compilation of techniques I have used successfully to deal with a current attack, warding off a coming attack, and finally, what to do in between when you feel just plain lousy. Many books shower you with so much information you don't know where to begin, it creates too much confusion in the mind and the book collects dust with all the other offending self helps. But the Survival Kit is there because I know you need immediate answers just like I did. I know how desperate you feel searching them out, and once found, how immediate you want the results you deserve. Anxiety is no joke, people might wonder what all the fuss is about. They think a little tension. But it's real, it hurts so bad inside you feel as though you're going to drop dead any second, but you won't. I'm still here to tell the tale, and so will you.

Find the Survival Kit and use straight away if you need to, it's there whenever despair envelopes you and help is urgently required.

'Survival Kit, turn to chapter 26'

Fear of admitting?

Been there, done that, and oh so bought the T-shirt. It's hard enough admitting to yourself you have a problem. Psychological problems bring with it big fears that other people are going to regard you as some sort of crazy nut. Thoughts such as, they might not like you, or, you might lose your job, are perfectly normal. Because you don't want to admit to them you have an ailment such as anxiety, fearing they'll drop you like a hot potato and move on to someone they regard as sane.

Just have a little faith in human kind. Stress related problems are now the most common reason why people have days off work, unable to cope with modern day living. So don't feel bad about it. Everybody suffers panic from one degree to another every day. By standing up and saying you have a problem, will help you come to terms with what you are going through and battle with this that much better.

I fought with it inside of me for too long, and later, the fear something was wrong had been fanned that many times, it was raging uncontrollably with no signs of dying down. Yet by telling people, I soon found in most cases it brought with it understanding and some compassion. It made me feel better other people knew. So if I had to run and hide, they understood the reasons why. I needn't go through all that fear, telling them during an attack why I felt the way I did, which only made matters worse. They knew, accepted the fact, and released the pressure. That's how it should be. Not the other way round.

'You need to diminish all stressful situations that heighten panic. The act of telling people helps remove worry if an attack should occur.'

Getting started

This can be frightening in itself. Thoughts of, 'will this work? What next if it doesn't work? I have nothing else to try. Will I feel like this forever? What's going to happen to me? I'm too scared to begin. I can't concentrate. I feel so ill how can I do this? What's happening? Maybe when I feel slightly better then I'll give it a try.'

Sound familiar? I had such thoughts. It's not uncommon to fear the unknown. From day to day we all experience such anguish, but where we're concerned, namely panic attack sufferers, it has become heightened. I had thoughts like; 'Why bother? You won't be around for much longer.'

Sounds awful doesn't it, but I had become so convinced I was going to die, it affected my work. People would call me and book their car in for a valet, normally for during the following week, and I'd say yes. But the voice in my head would say if you're still here. I mean, if I was alive. And the reasons I had were purely based upon how my body was reacting to stress, or more specifically, stressful thoughts.

So when starting your own recovery, instead of thinking why it won't work, go in with an open mind and give one hundred percent. I'm not saying you have to slog so hard you raise anxiety levels because the adrenaline is pumping. Just take your time. - If after ten minutes you need a rest, then take it. Or start tomorrow. Or the day after. But gradually you'll increase the time at your own pace, and that's the key. Getting a feel for how far you can safely go without bringing on the anxiety extends your confidence. And with more confidence, comes a longer period in which an attack is unlikely to happen for you.

But please, whatever you do, don't go beating yourself up over all of this. You went and bought this book, which is an achievement in itself, many people deny they have a problem such as this. Instead they choose to hide behind a chirpy, happy go lucky face, trying desperately to deal with numerous horrors buried beneath. But you're different. You have recognised the fact and want help, making it a first major step towards recovery.

And this shouldn't be underestimated. On its own, this can bring the emotions flowing, so start getting used to the feeling of a new beginning. Your body has probably been in this state for some time now, and any alteration to your immediate world may bring feelings of anxiety, accompanied by despondency and tearfulness. Hurtful memories might pass in and out, dragging you down further, taking you back to the comfort zone. The very same place you hate with all your heart but are fearful in leaving. Like a childhood security blanket. You know how it will feel and you draw comfort from it. Yet in this case, the fear of feeling normal is too much. Having to deal with normal world things can easily push you back, and panic rears its ugly head time and time again as some form of protection. But now it's outstayed its welcome, and we need to deal with it in one form or another.

'If you are willing, your life can, and will be about to change.'

Summary

Tick

Box

☐Try reading the entire book before attempting the exercises.

☐Use the *'Survival Kit'* whenever you need it.

☐Read chapter 17 on coping strategies.

☐Don't feel bad about anxiety, inform others to reduce stress.

☐Try and feel optimistic about the future and your recovery.

☐Keep taking your Rescue Remedy.

☐Remember, 'YOU ARE SAFE.'

☟Remedy Watch

Throughout this book you will notice the appropriate Bach flower remedies to take have been included when dealing with a particular emotion. This serves as a quick reference so you needn't go searching for the answer.

- 3 -

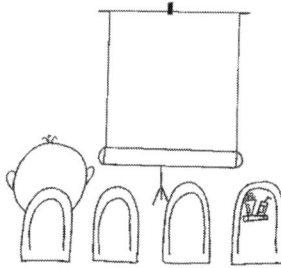

Introduction

Looking back over the past few years, I'll say panic disorder was probably the worst thing, and probably the best thing that's ever happened for me.

But wait, something is either good, or bad. How can it be possibly be both? That's just crazy. - Isn't it?

Well no. Because it meant I suffered for years, often painfully. Although I can't say I'd like to start over again just for the experience, I'm not a masochist. But I can honestly say it has changed my life for the better. It's opened me up, pulled my head out of the sand and kicked me into action. Otherwise I'd still be dreaming of becoming a writer and never actually achieving anything.

I'd already given up on inventing. Many ideas had gone to the wall, and money lost, and there was I floating in no man's land hoping something might fall in my lap one day, omitting the need to keep cleaning people's cars. Yet the fact was, I was always cleaning, and when I wasn't, I felt guilty, which meant what I really wanted to do stayed firmly fixed on the backburner. Next, add in a whole bucket full of self doubt mixed with a dollop of self hatred, and now the picture's looking more gloomy than a British seaside resort in the mid of winter.

So there is a positive to panic attacks, and they shouldn't necessarily be viewed as a bad thing. The fight or flight response is the science behind such attacks, but as the underlying reason which acts as a trigger becomes more complex, it's still telling you, me, and anyone else, it's time for change.

Yes you read that right, change. Anxiety attacks act as a wakeup call. To say finally, 'hey what's going on here? Why do I feel so lousy? What do I need to change? And where do I want to go from here?

Forget all that crap people have imposed over the years and stick two fingers up to the norm. Who wants regrets? Who wants to be saying in their twilight years, 'Of course dear, you know I could have done all that if I had wanted to.'

For me, I just don't want to be finding myself saying that, and feeling disappointment in myself for never doing what's in my heart. I see too many people doing this, and it fills me with great sadness for them. Some aren't on their death beds either, but they have given up for one reason or another, which is sad, especially when they have so much to offer and could make such a difference in the big wide world.

Presented the chance, most of us want to leave behind some kind of mark. A bit of something to remember us by when we're gone, whether it's world changing or more vicinity located; the result's the same. Dreams make us, without them we become the walking dead, lifeless beings who roam the planet wondering what the next installment of EastEnders or any other soap will bring. We care less for humanity and become so wrapped up in our portion of life we veg out, before eventually turning back into dust in a place where nobody remembers we existed.

But dreams on the other hand are great. You should never lose sight, and regularly participate in a bit of day dreaming to make sure of this. Hold it, see it, feel what it might be like to live it. And whatever you do from now on, fight for it. Keep fighting doggedly, and as long as you protect that dream from destructive outer influences, sooner rather than later, it will be there for you. You just have to do one simple thing….BELIEVE.

'Self belief is real power. When this is there for you anything can be achieved.'

Say. *'I have all the power I need within me. I believe fully in myself and in whatever I choose.'*

It's hard I know. When you're feeling down, and hurting so bad it feels like the end is near, there's actually a personal message locked in there. I can't sit and write what that message is for you because I don't honestly know. Mine would be different from yours. Just like the lady who lives at the end of the street would be different from the gentleman who lives above the off license. There is no way of putting a finger on it and saying 'X' is the secret cure for everyone. We all have circumstances of varying difference which means you shall soon discover your own journey and find the true answer. Whether it's regret, anger, a loss of a loved one, self hate, working overly hard, or whatever, the path is yours to overcome.

Sounds frightening? Don't worry, with help you'll soon be coming to terms and changing your life for the better.

Finally

Although you'll find many areas to follow, I genuinely hope through my own experiences of this frightening disorder I've cut out the dead ends. The ones that probably aren't worth bothering with because their value is low to nonexistent. I didn't want you getting bogged down. Remedies are there to work, and if it's costing you money and they don't do what it says on the tin, then quite frankly you're wasting hard earned cash on nothing more than time wasting hindrance. I can say that because I myself have spent hundreds on Chinese medicines, and several others that promised so much, but the core remedies that would have cut to the chase are detailed here for you. Follow the process and you'll heal. But please, for your own sake, stick at it. Many people don't give this kind of work a fair chance and walk away disregarding it as rubbish, or mumbo jumbo. They don't see immediate results in the first week or coming months and quit. What they're failing to understand is the body takes time to clear out the rubbish. Refuse stinks at the best of times as you know, your body emotional refuse is little different. Get rid of the garbage and stand back and admire the empty space. See how beautiful it is, energies can easily pass through a clear space, but put blockages in the way and the obstructions cause pains along with emotional turmoil.

Of course rubbish will return, we can never stop that, but now you'll understand what's happening and you'll learn to ditch it straight away before any harm comes. Stuff happens, but it doesn't mean you have to hold onto it any longer.

Just a thought

Why write a guide on how to defeat panic attacks when there are so many others on the market already?

Good question. But surfing on Amazon the other day I noticed they were mostly written by doctors who specialised in the field. I personally have nothing against them, but don't you find when you're told by someone who has experienced what you are feeling, there is some reassurance to be had. If they did it, and lived to tell the tale, then 'I can sure do it' mentality comes into play here.

Undoubtedly, fuelling one's mind with this belief system puts you streets ahead of somebody who was told by a specialist. I mean, it's not as though you're not listening to them, because you are, only one part of your brain is thinking. 'How do you know? Have you ever felt like this.' Which can also have the effect of them over simplifying panic attacks and dealing a possible cure, usually a few drug routes and a line such as, 'don't worry, it's just anxiety. Try to relax.'

They are good at the theory. And often their books supply many case studies with facts that are of no use and don't particularly make interesting reading. Especially when you're in such a state and you want help now, and don't care about the percentage of the population who suffer from attacks. They fail to grasp what's really going on.

The core. Like how trapped you feel. Or, how detached you've become even though you happen to be sitting amongst a crowd of noisy people. You know, the real life problems that create complex whirling emotions that need addressing before you momentarily spiral out of control. - These people don't know this. They can only write what they think it might be like, and then come up with a possible cure that doesn't really stop what you're feeling. It might make a difference, as they are drawing on therapy techniques which have been researched and proven to make a partial difference, but cure. No. You need a little extra help, which is why I was so compelled to write this book for you in the first place.

The bottom line is, if you want to get better read this book and act on it, if not, read a doctor's and get just more facts.

Summary

Tick

Box

☐Time for change in your life.

☐Hold onto your dreams.

☐Prepare to clear out the rubbish.

☐Follow my lead.

☐Remember, 'YOU ARE SAFE.'

- 4 -

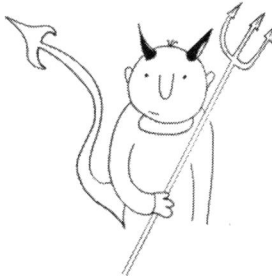

Hell Bound

The day my earth shook

Before we continue, I want to cover old ground with you here and now. I want to tell you about my first full blown panic attack that changed my life, so you needn't be worried anymore. So you can see the sensations you feel are no different to the ones I felt, and that there is nothing wrong with you. Your body reacts as it should when a perceived threat occurs, which means you are working fully, you just need to reclaim control and the outside world will turn from a place that scares you, to a world of endless possibilities.

But first let us travel back in time. Let me take you to a period when I thought I was just going to have a normal night out, but it soon changed into something I couldn't have imagined possible, and in truth, never knew my body could react the way it did. This was my new beginning.

The Cinema

Sitting there my throat began to tighten, a sensation I hate. I tried to ignore what was happening at first and just concentrate on the film, but that didn't last long. The sensation got stronger and my breath started to feel restricted.

'Okay,' I thought, 'I can handle this.' But in truth, I couldn't. My heart fluttered, my chest tightened, and I began to sweat. The cold sweat of fear trickled down my back and now things felt more serious than ever before.

'What's happening?' I questioned myself. 'Am I dying?'

I slowly scanned the cinema and started to stare at the people seated beside me. I wondered if they'd mind I had to get past. Then I made all kinds of reasons for staying. The film had twenty minutes left to run, surely I could stay, last it out and no one would be the wiser.

There were two fears at work here. One, the fear of dying, and two, dying in front of all those people. I had strong images of myself clutching my heart, pleading for help, then collapsing and dying in horrible, unbearable pain.

I stood up, said something to my brother like, 'got to go outside for a moment' which he interpreted as I needed the toilet.

A moment later I'd passed all the cinema goers and was heading into the foyer. It seemed quiet there, which suited me fine as I was convinced my seconds were numbered, and anyway, I couldn't bear people looking at me.

I pushed the large entrance doors of the cinema and walked out into the cool fresh air of the night. Normally this would have been a nice experience, especially after the hot cinema, but my throat was still tight and I found myself fighting for breath.

Legs resembling jelly, I headed towards the arcade come bowling alley, for I knew there was a bar there and I'd be able to get some water.

The building was bustling with life. Machines sung laser blasts as people killed aliens, a low thud from a punch bag on the boxing machine accompanied by screaming car engines in a virtual grand prix. All in all, it was a typical night in Norwich.

Slightly light headed, I made for the bar where a pretty young girl was busily drying some glasses. I caught her attention and asked for some water, which she kindly obliged filling a mug from the kitchen. I smiled and thanked her before taking a sip.

The water slipped down easily, but had little effect, all I could feel was the symptoms intensifying, yet I was sure these feelings were hardly symptoms, I was going to die. I was actually going to die.

Next I began looking for someone, someone who'd be able to help, who I'd be happy to ask. - I couldn't see anyone. I walked back towards the door but had second thoughts and looked a little harder, but still nothing. My legs where growing so weak I was having trouble standing, my stomach had cramped worse than ever before, and my chest tightened to what felt like bursting point.

Back towards the exit a man asked me if I was okay. He was a security guard. But before he used to serve me at an electronics supplier in the city. If I close my eyes I can remember the conversation.

'You alright mate?' Asked the guard.

'I can't breathe,' I said softly.

'Come outside and get some fresh air, you'll feel better.'

I tried to breathe and talk, but it came rather muted. 'My chest, it hurts. It's so tight.'

The guard looked at me suspiciously, 'you been drinking?'

'No,' I replied, 'only water.'

I stagger and he catches me. 'Do you want an ambulance?'

I stare at him, scared and unsure what to do. -'I don't know,' I said finally. 'Maybe. – Yes, I think so.'

My brother Stuart turned up at this point, the film had finished and it soon became evident I hadn't left to go to the gentleman's.

'I'm his brother, what's going on?'

The guard stepped forward. 'He's complaining of chest pains, don't worry, an ambulance has been called already.'

Stuart sat me down on a concrete block, but it soon became obvious I was getting worse. I started swearing really bad, to the point couples stared momentarily and rushed past. One man grabbed his horrified girlfriend by the arm, and pulled her into the nearby bar, probably thinking I was either crazy, or on drugs. - And that's when it hit me. – I was alone. Totally, utterly, alone. A feeling so intense, it breached terror. There was me, my throbbing heart, and an expanse of nothingness beyond.

While my memory becomes a little fuzzy here, I think a man asked my brother if I was alright. Stuart said everything was under control, and the concerned passerby gave a slight nod and departed. But the point being, someone had asked. One of the public was worried and that was enough to bring me round and start to fight. - I needed a bag. A paper one. I can't recall why. Probably something my dad had said once to cure hyperventilation, but I gasped for a bag. Somehow I relayed this to the guards and my brother, and what followed next was a sudden rush of activity, while a grand search commenced. I heard people shouting, running, slamming of doors, when all of a sudden thrust into my hands was the object of my desire. A large popcorn bag.

A minute later, I looked at Stuart and forced a weak smile. 'I can feel my hand. It's coming back.' I clenched my hand and unclenched it a couple of times, wondering in the marvel. Yet at the time, I didn't think I'd feel anything but numbness again. I was returning. I, Richard, was coming alive.

Stuart forced the bag back over my mouth, 'Shut up and keep breathing.' It seemed almost comical, but neither of us were laughing.

All of a sudden the sirens and blue flashing lights of a speeding ambulance appeared on the scene. Two dark haired paramedics jumped out from the cab, and came rushing over with a green bag full of all kinds of goodies.

'You alright mate?' Asked the driver.

I nodded, 'I'm getting feeling back.' I felt so tired by now I wanted to rest, but instead they put me in the back of the ambulance for a check over.

I shook violently. No matter how hard I tried, I couldn't stay still with all that adrenaline rushing around my system. I sat bent over, trying to relieve the ache in my stomach while listening to the paramedic.

'Just tell me what happened?' He asked.

I rattled off the story in double time, but by the lack of activity I guessed there was nothing to worry about.

'Sounds to me you've just suffered a panic attack, there's no obstruction in the throat area and you seem perfectly fine now.' The other medic who'd just taken a seat by his colleague agreed.

I could have cried. The emotions were high, one moment I thought I was about to die, and then I'm told there's nothing wrong with me. But something had happened that night, something felt wrong, and although they gave me a clean bill of health, I was scared of it happening again, and then I wouldn't be so lucky.

'So what happens now? Should I carry the bag from now on?' I said.

'Might be a good idea, just until you get over this' said the second paramedic. 'It's not going to harm.'

'I disagree.' The first medic glanced at his colleague before returning his gaze back to me. 'You need to deal with the problem, that's the only way you'll overcome this.'

I wasn't so sure at the time. I looked down at the tatty popcorn bag in my right hand, and whenever I thought of leaving it behind, my heart would pick up and the anxiety built again.

'I'll keep it for now,' I decided.

But the first medic hadn't liked my response. 'You don't want to have to carry that around for the rest of your life, do you?'

I felt panic, I felt pain, I wanted to run. I didn't want confrontation. I never wanted any of this.

'Because that's what's going to happen if you carry the bag around all the time,' he concluded.

It became harder, so I agreed. I backed down. I backed down like

I'd always done in a fight to keep the peace. But still, when I stepped from the ambulance and thanked the both of them, the bag stayed with me. I just couldn't let it go.

The ambulance started and disappeared into the night, leaving my brother and I standing alone. A couple of the guards came by with their hand to their ear, FBI style, and didn't seem bothered I'd made it through. I kind of wondered later if they'd reacted differently if I had died that night, but deep down I'm glad that point was never discovered. For me, the attack was over, and that's all that mattered.

Where did that leave me exactly? Although I disagreed at the time, the first paramedic was right. Carrying something, rather like a comfort blanket, is walking on dangerous ground. Suppose I forgot the bag one day, and on remembering, I had a major attack. Like Walt Disney's Dumbo and the feather. When Dumbo held the feather in his trunk he could fly because that's what he was led to believe. But when the feather fell from poor Dumbo's trunk, the belief had gone. He was heading for ground at terrific speed, and it wasn't until his friend told him the feather was bogus; holding no magical power whatsoever, the predicament became resolved. Dumbo believed he had the power, and because he believed, he flew again.

By dealing with it, like the paramedic had said, the problem would eventually leave, alleviating the use of a tool such as the paper bag. The bag would signify safety. Decreasing the chance of any more violent attacks, as its very presence bought peace of mind. Just as sufferers have spoken of a particular room where they feel safe. It isn't the room itself that's stops the panic, it's the belief the room stops the panic, that stops the panic. Just as the feather in Dumbo's case made him fly, because he believed it would make him fly. Panic doesn't become an issue when we decide it isn't one anymore. Both scenarios are the same.

Belief along with understanding helps us overcome fear. I had to find that out the hard way. But when you're so low, so ill, and you just want it all to go away, I'm afraid negative is easier than positive. Everything becomes too much and this in itself becomes a downward spiral.

Summary

Tick

Box

☐My first full blown panic attack was a wake-up call. I needed to change my way of thinking.

☐The sensations I felt are no different to the ones you are feeling.

☐There is nothing wrong with you, this is a natural response to a perceived danger.

☐Belief along with understanding helps us overcome fear.

☐My own journey unraveled the mysteries of panic attacks. I can help you through yours.

☐You can regain control, panic will soon be a thing of the past.

☐Remember, 'YOU ARE SAFE.'

- 5 -

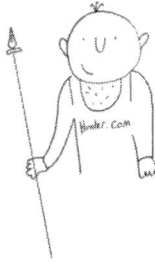

So what is a Panic Attack?

The basis of a panic attack comes from what we call the fight or flight response. It originates from the days when primitive humans lived in caves, hunted wild animals for food, and needed something a bit special when danger loomed. It's a response for survival, pure and simple.

But let's get more detail. To explain the mechanics I shall enlist the help of Ug, a Neolithic man, along with his wife, the most beautiful, delectable, Dorithia.

Now Ug is a true hunter, he is muscular, powerful, and knows how to swing a club to his advantage. You just wouldn't want to mess with him in any shape or form.

Beautiful Dorithia on the other hand is slim and petite. She's also the finest gourmet cook around and looks after their new born Ug junior.

As you can clearly see, Ug and Dorithia possess completely different roles within the family unit. But man or woman, it doesn't matter, both own the natural response due to the simple fact wild animals aren't picky when it comes to food. For today however, it is Ug we shall concentrate on, as he's presently out in the field hiding behind a convenient boulder rock.

There he is, spying over the top so not to be seen. Ug has just spotted a fine woolly mammoth. His eyes now zero in. All concentration is taken up by this wild powerful beast, because he knows once killed, his family needn't go without for the soon cold winter months.

Ug reaches for his weapons of choice. A tall spear accompanied by a hefty knobbed club. He's moving stealthily, keeping low while out of the mammoths limited sight so not to alert his presence.

Closing in, he slowly prepares his spear by lifting it high. Like a javelin thrower at the games, he gives it all he's got, and the long shaft cuts through the air at great speed, striking the beast squarely in the side. The mammoth raises its head towards the blue sky, and resonates a loud cry of pain.

Wounded, the mammoth is trying to run, but the blood loss is weakening its energy. Ug is cunning here, instead of risking his life and fighting such tonnage, he waits a couple of hours to find the animal further up the trail. Except by now, it's collapsed on its side utterly exhausted.

Ug, obviously feeling rather pleased with himself, is moving in to finish the job off. But wait! What's this? Ug is no longer alone. There are other living things out there that will steal his kill given half the chance. In this case, a big sabre tooth tiger with an awful temper has just emerged from seemingly nowhere.

Ug stops dead, he's standing like stone, hoping the tiger hasn't seen his kill. But it has, and now it's licking its lips almost tasting the juicy red meat.

This doesn't look good. Its deadly long claws have extended and it's beginning to run towards Ug. It will kill Ug if it has to for the prize.

Ug's eyes open wide and he takes a single gulp. His Neolithic brain, although slightly more primitive than ours, is working out whether to stand and fight, or run.

Without conscious thought, Ug's body is preparing itself.

His heart begins to pound, transporting oxygen-carrying blood to the parts that need it. Breathing rate increases. Oxygen is required by muscles to help transform sugar into energy. Ug's senses this as sight and hearing are enhanced. Blood is diverted from non essential areas so Ug appears pale. He's suddenly sick to lighten the load. Sweat is becoming more apparent as his body tries to cool down from the exertion.

Ug is now experiencing the *'Fight or Flight Response.'*

It would be stupid of him to stand and fight such a threatening animal, so instead, he's just turned on the spot. Crouching, so as to look as least threatening as possible, yet still watching the Sabre's every move.

The sabre slows, circling the kill, he gently muzzles the mammoths rear quarter, but eyes are fixed on Ug. For the cat, Ug is too much of a threat, and in one giant pounce the tiger makes for him.

Like a sprinter out of the blocks Ug's running as fast as he can. The dust is being kicked up behind him, and he crosses the open space in a shorter time than even he thought ever possible.

Back at the kill, the sabre's showing little interest in following. He licks his nose and turns around. He eyes the dying beast a few feet away and casually saunters over. Ug is nowhere to be seen. The hunt is truly over.

And to us, it appears Ug has found super human powers to avoid danger, but really his body has upped its own natural strength for a short period of time. Had it not, he wouldn't have made it back to the cave and be enjoying one of his wife's specialties, lizard and snail soup with rock dust seasoning and a side salad.

So that was way back then. Why do we need it now?

That's the million dollar question isn't it. Why in our modern day lives do we need such a response? Because, although we don't come up against drooling sabre tooth tigers anymore, we can find ourselves in dangerous situations where a response can be useful. People have shown great strength in the past. For instance, I can recall a man finding super human power to turn a car over where the driver had become trapped. Normally the man would never even think he could achieve such a feat, so had it not been for the fight or flight response, the task would have been impossible.

But that doesn't help you. You see, your response is being triggered by every little situation, and the more fear you bring into that panic attack, the worse the sensations become. *(See panic loop on next page)*. That's how it becomes when the system has become oversensitive. But fear not, fight or flight can be de-sensitized, and you can live without panic once more.

Break the *Panic Loop* = Break the Anxiety

THE MODERN DAY PANIC LOOP

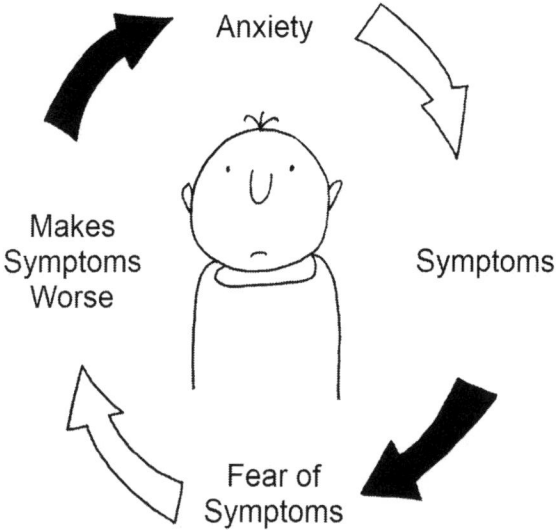

Anxiety

Makes
Symptoms
Worse

Symptoms

Fear of
Symptoms

After all, what is **Fear** anyway?
False **E**vidence **A**ppearing **R**eal

Summary

Tick

Box

☐ Panic attacks are what we call the *'Fight or Flight Response.'* It's our response for survival.

☐ The slightest of fears currently drive the response.

☐ You can de-sensitize and live a normal life again.

☐ Remember, 'YOU ARE SAFE.'

- 6 -

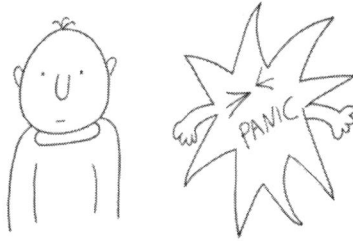

Why does Panic Come???

The more I wrote this book for you, the more I came to realise the underlying factors why we as human beings subconsciously call upon panic. After all, we are all flesh and blood from the human mould. We all have the same emotions, although some choose to ignore them, or are frightened to express them, yet the initial programming remains the same for every one of us. In short, we react the same way when dealing with fear. But that's not the whole story, it is my belief we all get to the final stage, namely panic attacks, via the same route. I say that, because by talking to people I've learnt a lot about their hopes, fears, and hang-ups, which all point to panic in various degrees. From mild, where the person has simply lost direction, seems disinterested in virtually everything and can't seem to get a grip with life, to the raging horror and utter fear of all imaginable when attacks become more of a problem. These paralyzing fears are what stops us in our tracks, leaving us unable to move because we fear the worst is going to strike. Our bodies are in turmoil, our minds race from one terrifying thought to another, and worse still, we seem to have no control over the thoughts, feelings, and physical symptoms that plague us. But that is the trick of panic, in fact we do have control, it's just our bodies are making us believe we don't have the power to stop this from happening.

But firstly, let's have a look at the kind of challenges that appear.

The common reasons panic attacks strike:

○Not listening to what your body is trying to tell you. You feel tired, stomach discomfort, light headed, shaky, sickness etc.

○Find it hard to switch off. Your mind doesn't switch off when your body does.

○Feeling uncomfortable with people. A sense of loneliness. Worried what other people may think of you.

○Fear of rejection. Always trying to please everybody all of the time.

○Known fears, e.g. dentist, getting on a train, a visit to the cinema.

○Lack of confidence. Not trusting yourself.

○Feeling you're not in control of your life.

○Not being able to cope with simple tasks.

○Living/working in an unhappy environment, or within an unhappy relationship.

○Money worries. Will I have enough to pay the bills?

○Loneliness. Fear of being alone and a fear of being alone and ill.

○Feelings of abandonment.

○ Fear of the Fear.

○ Knowing you deserve better, but not knowing how to change.

○ Repeatedly berating yourself. Anger towards yourself and others.

○ Feelings of being overwhelmed. Everything seems worse or harder than it actually is.

○ Inability to control racing thoughts. Feel as though you are bogged down and going nowhere fast.

○ Feeling cross with yourself because you didn't go with your own personal gut feeling.

○ You base yourself on what others think and expect of you.

○ Emotionally you feel out of control, leading to 'am I going crazy' thinking.

○ You feel you've been kicked so hard in the past it has led to 'What's the point?' thinking.

○ A strong sense you don't belong. - In the lowest you feel unworthy. A screw up, useless, a waste of space, possibly thoughts of suicide as well.

○ Then a big one, you think you've got some terrible illness.

Do any of these sound familiar?

From personal experience, I can relate to every one of those above, and you might recognise them straight off also, but it's nice to know these emotions are not yours alone. There are other people out there who feel exactly the same as you do right now, and just by recognising this, it can be a moment of relief in itself.

'The list is universal; it's the way we respond that makes the difference.'

They are painful though, and I don't think any should be taken lightly. To the sufferer it feels as though hope is all lost, you sink inside, your mind rattles through thoughts such as beating yourself up, or asking why me. Anger is a player too. You feel an outcast, lonely, and have a strong belief there is nobody out there who can help. But I hope from reading this book you have realised you are not alone, and panic can be beaten. These emotions can be brought under control so they aren't troublesome anymore.

Reprogramming with positive takes the pain away, the dirty black cloud that's been hovering just above your head can be changed into a beautiful rainbow of opportunity, it all begins with a single thought. – Let's now look at the positive.

○You don't have to feel like this.

○Life doesn't have to be this way.

○Panic is your body's reaction to your way of thinking. You can change it around.

○Once you clear all these negative emotions out of the way, you will begin to find yourself, and then anything is possible.

○A feeling of peace and well-being will come.

Panic is curable, and although you probably don't feel like it now, later you will start to look at your life and where it's heading. Life will start to look like an opportunity to do something fantastic, instead of the gloomy picture you are holding right now. Don't get me wrong, I know how it feels. Tomorrow seems too much. Heck, the next hour feels a struggle in survival, let alone thinking about the rest of your life!

Why is that? - Because the pain, sickness, and sheer horror of panic has swept over you with such force, you can't see anything else apart from the pain and confusion you are in. You're convinced there is something wrong with you, that something will strike you down any moment, and it's just a matter of when. Your mind replays different scenarios. Yet without realising, you are actually fuelling the panic further. The more destructive thoughts you have, the adrenaline goes up, and the body reacts accordingly.

I'm not saying it's easy to change, it does take time and effort, but there is some satisfaction to be had when you conquer each hurdle. Gradually, you will feel better for all of this, and when the days come when panic isn't a problem anymore, you'll feel on top of the world.

Summary

Tick

Box

☐From human to human our emotions are the same.

☐You don't have to feel like this anymore.

☐It takes time, you can lead a panic free life once more.

☐What you are feeling is perfectly normal for someone in an anxiety state. I will help you get through this.

☐The world can be your oyster. You will regain control over this.

☐Remember, 'YOU ARE SAFE.'

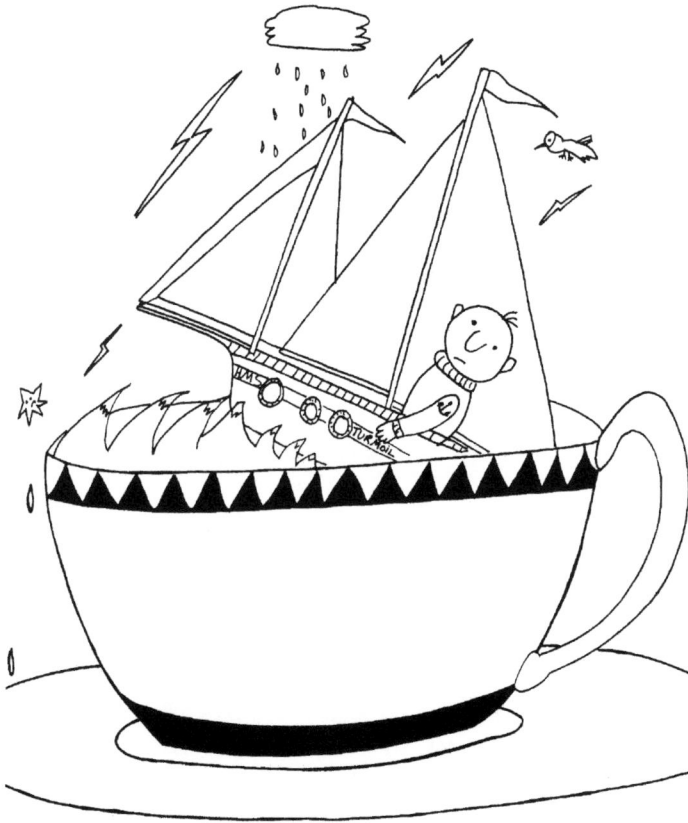

Storm in a Tea Cup

When we blow things out of proportion the problems become so big we invite panic and anxiety. By realising this, and not allowing things to have an effect on us, we can beat this.

- 7 -

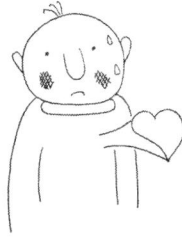

Sensations & Dealing with the Mental Side

'Note: It's vital you see your doctor for a check-up, to eliminate any other possible medical condition(s) other than anxiety.'

When you experience these terrifying thoughts and feelings for the first time it's likely you are going to either end up in A&E, or at your doctors. Understandably it's very upsetting, it feels like your whole world has just crashed down, and the thoughts often rotate around maybe you are suffering from some horrible life threatening disease. I've lost count how many times I've ended up visiting the doctor, or hospital, in a state of fear, only to be turned back with a clean bill of health. I've been put on the ECG machine and had blood tests more times than I can remember. And although this gives a moment of relief, you find yourself convinced perhaps your doctor might have missed something because the anxiety attacks keep on happening. – And in truth, no matter how frightening the symptoms are, the mental side of this disorder is probably more challenging to deal with than the physical side. After all, anxiety is a mental disorder, the physical feelings are just a byproduct of a mindset firmly stuck in fear. But this can be changed, and when it does, the feelings disappear.

But for now, you find it difficult to get the bad thoughts out of your head, real negative thoughts about what your body is doing inside, and you soon become fixated on every little twitch and pain that is happening within. And the more you pay attention to these symptoms, the more fear you are injecting into them, creating a barrage of physical feelings that only get worse and appear with higher regularity.

What does this all mean? - You are starting to become over-sensitised. And the more fear you put into an already fearful state, you are adding to the anxiety, and it can easily spiral out of control. And when this happens, it feels as though you are at the mercy of your own body and you seemingly have no power over it any more.

Yesterday you had control, today you feel like you as a person has been stripped away, and you will never be the same again. It's called 'Depersonalisation.' You feel you've lost something and you are left wandering around in a dream like state, the world and your life has become vague, happiness doesn't play a part in it anymore. Quite often you will hear people say, 'I used to be such a happy person, always laughing and joking, and now I can't feel the joy in anything anymore.' You feel like you are outside of your body and things around you are not quite real. – Again, that's depersonalisation. But please please remember this. And I want to make this clear to you because it is so important.

'You are not all alone with this; we all feel and think these horrible feelings, sensations, and mental thoughts. They are part of the condition. But if you can change how you respond to these symptoms, then you are well on your way

to recovery.'

What do I mean by this statement? Changing how you respond? In simple terms, don't read anything into them. Don't think, I am dying. Think, oh, I have a pain, or, I feel dizzy, and let it pass. – How can I possibly do that??? You say. Well, don't worry for now, because I will talk more on this along with coping strategies in a later chapter.

For now, let's have a look at the common symptoms that come with anxiety and panic attacks.

Symptoms:

O Muscle tension.

O Headaches.

O Dizziness.

O Shortness of breath.

O Tight chest.

O Chest pains.

O Electric shock like feelings.

O Sore chest.

O Tingling in centre of chest.

O Sharp pains all over the body.

O Sickness.

O Tiredness.

O Drowsiness.

O Feelings of being on the verge of passing out.

○ Pins and needles.

○ Dry mouth.

○ Palpitations.

○ Stomach ache.

○ Frequent trips to the toilet.

○ Difficulty sleeping.

○ A feeling like you are leaving your body.

○ A Sense of dread.

○ Difficulty concentrating.

○ The same negative thoughts going around your head, e.g. I am going to die, my heart is going to stop etc.

○ Irritability.

○ Impatience.

○ Easily distracted.

○ Deep sense of fear.

○ Unable to talk with anybody, inability to communicate.

○ Wanting to run and hide away.

○ Deep sense something is wrong.

○ A lump in your throat.

○ Every twinge means something else is wrong with you. (Health Anxiety).

○ Inability to form friendships, and lose the ones you had.

○ Find it hard to be sympathetic or help others.

○ Every little thing sends your body into shock.

○ Dry retching.

○ Unable to leave your house because of a strong fear something might happen to you.

○ Disconnected from society.

○ Repeated questioning why you are different.

○ Feelings that you can't cope.

○ Feelings of no joy, and that you will never feel happy and carefree.

○ Loneliness.

○ Depression.

○ Wanting a relationship with somebody who understands you.

○ Desire for help and support.

○ Shyness.

And it might surprise you these probably aren't all the symptoms either. And just because you don't see a symptom listed here you are currently dealing with, it doesn't mean there is something else wrong, because we all experience stress and anxiety in different ways. There is no common one set of feelings we all suffer with, although what we do feel, changes over time. But you will become stronger, and with my help, you will start to see these feelings subside and the real you begin to emerge. This has all happened for a reason, and the reason being to improve every aspect of your life.

So, let us now look at the more common symptoms in a bit more detail.

Muscle tension - Probably the first signs you are stressed come way of muscle tension. You can use this as an indication when relaxation is needed. Check for tension in the shoulders, neck area, and arms. By releasing tension this removes this symptom.

To counteract:

1. Take *Rescue Remedy* and *Rock Water.*

2. Write down all your worries. After, screw the piece of paper up and throw in bin.

3. Lie down; tense all your muscles for ten seconds and release. Do this three times. (Don't do this if you suffer from either a heart condition or high blood pressure).

4. Use the breathing technique for five minutes as described in the *'Survival Kit.'*

5. Have a hot bath. Add herbal bubble bath and relax in the warmth. You can also add *Rock Water* to float away stress. See *'Survival Kit.'*

6. Meditate with a good meditation tape. Half an hour to an hour should do the trick. After, flop into bed for a good night's sleep. Tomorrow you'll feel better.

7. Drink hot water with a slice of lemon in it

8. Changes take time, so be gentle on yourself. – Remember, what you are feeling are only the effects of Anxiety.

Headache -We all have headaches from time to time, but tension induced ones can last for days when stressed. Easily detected by the proximity, the upper forehead. Back of neck tends to be sore as well. You'll find most head pain comes from either tension in the neck muscles, related to your increased anxiety, or racing uncontrolled thoughts.

To counteract:

1. Gently massage the back of neck.

2. Use a wheat bag, or warm hot water bottle wrapped in a towel, and place over the sore neck area. Try gently rubbing your temples in a circular motion.

4. Lay down in a dimly lit room without a pillow, close your eyes and relax. Allow your mind to drift, see the images, and watch them gently go.

5. Imagine all the tension seeping from every pore of your body and flowing away. Breathe in relaxation, breathe out stress.

6. Write down all your thoughts. See *'Keeping a Diary.'*

Pains – These can be confusing because they not only vary in strength, but seem to change position from one minute to the next. Yet it's all caused by muscle spasm. - You know the ones in your chest that feel so tight and jiggle as though your heart's in trouble? Again, muscle spasm. They are disturbing and darn right uncomfortable, but with the knowledge of what they are, usually caused by tension and the effects of adrenaline, they seem less threatening.

Muscle spasm and muscle tension will plague you a lot of the time until you gain some kind of control. But I guarantee, as you improve so will these particular symptoms.

To counteract:

1. Be kinder to the self. Keep an eye on overworking and self berating.

---

2. Use relaxation techniques regularly. See, *'Visualisation & Survival Kit.'*

3. Eat regularly and the correct food. See, *'Diet & the Importance.'*

4. Say to yourself, *'there is nothing to fear, this is a symptom of anxiety and nothing else.'*

5. Take **Rescue Remedy.**

6. Drink hot water with a slice of lemon in it.

Breathing difficulty – Another scary one. Especially combined with what I've already discussed. But there is nothing wrong with you. This is just a sensation. The muscles in your chest area tighten, and although you feel you can't get a full breath, actually you can. It's very odd, but still nothing to worry about.

To counteract:

1. Relax. Take your mind away from the problem. Chatting to somebody helps, or watch a DVD.

2. Slow the breath and breathe deep into the tummy. The feeling will pass. **Rescue Remedy** will be of help here.

3. Keep reminding yourself there is nothing wrong, it is only anxiety.

Swallowing difficulty – Slightly more disturbing than the breathing, but ultimately, tension in the throat muscles involved in the swallowing process get tight, and you feel you can't swallow.

This symptom hits everybody, especially when in company, or when somebody is watching you. Again, there is no threat, it's purely psychologically activated.

> **To counteract:**
>
> 1. Desensitise. By gradually introducing yourself to situations that create panic, it trains the brain into thinking it can cope. Over time, you'll notice situations which were once a problem you can now breeze through. See, *'To Walk the Devil's Yard.'*
>
> 2. Use *Rescue Remedy*.
>
> 3. Have a hot drink.
>
> 4. Relax, get some rest.
>
> 5. Talk with a friend.

Dizziness – You feel a little light headed, yet you're unlikely to fall over because of this. After all, it wouldn't do to fall when a wild animal is running after you, and this is fight or flight response related. What's actually happening is the blood is being moved away from less vital organs and pumped to the muscles for work. It feels rather like you've been on a roller coaster ride and the blood hasn't made it fully back after the big dipper. There is nothing to worry about, as the panic attack subsides so will your dizziness.

Also, shallow breathing has this effect. If you were to hold your breath for any reasonable length of time, you'd feel a bit dizzy, right? Which is why it's so important to control the breath.

From a mental angle, try not to let the fear run away with you.

Because the more you feed the dizziness with worry and fear, the worse the symptom will become. So, however unpleasant this is, however close you feel to passing out, just allow the feeling to wash over you without reacting to the episode. The more practiced you become, and the more you concentrate on your breathing, not to mention making sure you have eaten something recently. (Low blood sugar). This shall pass.

To counteract:

1. Relaxation techniques. Sit down somewhere quiet, close your eyes and concentrate on the breath. Breathe deep into the tummy to the count of four, breath out to the count of four. – Use **Rescue Remedy**.

2. Eat something.

3. Don't react to the dizziness, let it pass without feeding it with fear. – Reassure yourself this is only anxiety.

4. Take a rest. Lie down and get some sleep.

5. Meditation.

The shakes – At one time or another you might have noticed your hands were shaking quite visibly when anxious. This is down to our old friend muscle tension again. Food starvation also has the same effect, because we start to run on adrenaline instead of energy given by our food. A blood sugar drop will bring anxiety like symptoms, so make sure you eat something regularly.

To counteract:

1. Have something to **eat**. (Low blood Sugar). We burn a lot more energy in an anxious state so keep the meals small but often. **Muesli bars** are especially good when on the run. See **'Diet & the Importance.'**

2. Relax. Meditate.

3. Use **Rescue Remedy**.

---

4. Be easier on yourself.

5. Stop rushing and take regular time outs.

Stomach discomfort – Indigestion can build so high you convince yourself you really are going to have a heart attack. Pressure in the chest, heart burn, all make you think the worst. But it's wind created from anxiety, kicking off the kidneys to produce the adrenaline which creates the acid. You'll probably feel sick as well. The fight or flight demands an evacuation of the stomach to lighten the load for running, and it just so happens acid does this nicely.

Another discomfort is more abdominal, where the gut muscles are affected by stress (more adrenaline), which speeds up the wave of contractions which move our food along. This has the effect of the contents entering the last part of the bowl, the rectum, too fast.

Where normally the water is absorbed here and the liquid turns to solid, that doesn't happen. Instead we get the familiar feeling of diarrhea, and a trip to the nearest toilet can be quite imminent. Then we have what's known as I.B.S, or irritable bowel syndrome. Where it differs from diarrhea, is this strikes without warning. Stomach cramps leading to sudden explosion of liquid. This can be quite violent at times and extremely painful. Some foods may have the same effect, because you might have an intolerance, so it pays to steer clear of these. What's not so easy to steer clear of are situations where stress occurs, and as I.B.S is caused primarily by stress, you'll find when the panic attacks become more controlled, so will this particular problem.

Remove the *Fear* = Better Digestion

To counteract:

1. Eat and drink sensibly, take nothing that will upset your stomach. See chapter, *'Diet and the Importance'*, for more on I.B.S.

2. Try not to get over tired. The symptoms tend to worsen when exhausted.

3. Relax. Take note how you are holding your abdomen. When stressed we tend to hold our stomach under tension, tense these muscles, and release, check regularly.

4. When in trouble, use a reputable diarrhea elimination tablet. Although a last resort, it can save you when particularly bad.

5. Carry around indigestion tablets, again they can save you when wind becomes too much of a problem to cope.

6. Rest. Use the *Rescue Remedy.*

7. Drink plenty of still water to flush the system and replenish fluids. Also try boiled water with a slice of lemon to calm an acidy stomach and counteract the flight or fight response.

8. Anxiety elimination removes the symptom.

9. Remember this is just anxiety.

'Irritable bowel is very much a symptom of anxiety, not a disease.'

Fatigue – You sleep, but when waking you're as tired as when you went to bed the previous night. - Are you sore? I mean, when you wake, do your muscles feel sore and tender when touched? If yes, then you haven't been resting as well as you first thought.

When we are in an anxious state our muscles are working overtime. Basically, they need more energy to do this, and while we can put up with this for a surprisingly long time, sooner or later everything gets on top of us. We need rest. Although with panic in such a heightened state, rest seems unlikely, it is essential to try and relax.

But there's physical tiredness, and there's mental tiredness. Physical comes as mentioned. But mental, is because our thoughts are racing all the time. Our brains need a rest at some point, but you're not letting it, all that worry is having an effect. Both together, and this symptom turns into excessive fatigue, where everything becomes too much to handle. In this state, we tend to get quite overwhelmed, and feel negative about ourselves and other people. We also feel unable to cope with what can be seemingly simple tasks.

To counteract:

1. Take more rests throughout the day, slow the body down from all that rush rush.

2. Plan the day out realistically and do no more. Bring structure in as best you can. *'You can't get stressed about not doing work you hadn't planned that day.'*

3. Make time to relax at the end of the day. Unwinding is very important, just like the warm down is for an athlete who's just run a marathon.

4. Don't gobble your food down, take your time and make it much more of an event.

5. Write down your thoughts. See, *'Keeping a Diary.'*

6. Try and calm the mind. Distract yourself from your worries.

7. Breathe in relaxation, breathe out stress. Imagine white light entering on the in breath, and dirty black light exiting on the out breath. - Look after yourself.

Palpitations/Chest pain – These are rapid heartbeats, or more likely, a series of extra beats each followed by a pause, a space where the early beat should have been, making it seem as if the heart has an irregular rate. This is a horrible sensation and leads you onto thoughts of, 'oh my God, something is seriously wrong. I'm going to have a heart attack.'

Yet this couldn't be further from the truth. It's actually caused by the direct action of adrenaline on the heart, and as such, is a physical aspect of your anxiety. There is nothing wrong with your heart, you are producing too much adrenaline and it's running on super fuel. So as frightening as palpitations are, they do no harm. The trick is to recognise when they strike, relax as best you can, and wait for them to pass.

To counteract:

1. Use the breathing technique, control the breath and lower your anxiety.

2. Use the **Rescue Remedy** every ten minutes.

3. Say to yourself, *'this is only a symptom of my anxiety, there is nothing wrong with me.'*

4. Try and relax. Sleep is very good. Watch a film, listen to some music, or perhaps talk to somebody to distract from what's going on inside.

5. Talk positive to yourself. Keep reminding yourself this will pass.

> 6. Eat something, your blood sugar might have dropped causing this symptom.

Sweating/Hot flush/Sweaty palms/Temperature changes – This is to cool the body down, everything's running fast preparing you to run away from that nasty animal out on the plain, so it's no surprise heat is going to be a factor here. You are fine, reduce the anxiety by telling yourself you're okay, and there is nothing to worry about. This is only a symptom of anxiety. It will pass.

> **To counteract:**
>
> 1. Breathe correctly to calm the body.
>
> 2. Drink plenty of still water. *(2 Litres RDA)**
>
> 3. Again relax. You are coming to no harm.
>
> 4. Take Rescue Remedy every ten minutes.

* RDA = Recommended daily dosage.

So there we have it, some of the symptoms we have to deal with, but some of them are so terrifying they send you into even more panic. So what can you do? For me, I found the sharp pains in the chest and tightness the worst sensation, closely followed by dizziness, and not to mention the barrage of negative thoughts. In the moment it is very hard to deal with and it only enforces all the negative thoughts, making panic and anxiety worse and longer lingering. But you can overcome these symptoms by learning how to feel without reaction. By saying to yourself 'Ouch, that really hurts,' then concentrating on what you are doing, whether its washing the dishes, or talking to a loved one, ignore the symptom as best you can. And when you do this, it will just give up and fall away. Say, 'okay do your worst,' challenge the feeling, and what you'll see is the sensation disappear.

Why does this work? Because you have taken the fear from the situation. Anxiety feeds on fear, take away the fear, and the symptoms can no longer exist. Of course they will return time and time again, your body has got into a habit, but eventually your brain will realise it doesn't need to do this anymore, and you will start to notice the sensations gradually get less and less frequent. When you see this happen, your mind will automatically swap concentration from what's going on inside of you, and move to more what is going on the outside of you. - The rewiring of your brains neurons has begun. The longer you reinforce this pattern, this habit will break, and you'll find your confidence will eventually grow.

And that's the key, when your confidence grows, you'll be able to cope with life knowing your body is not going to turn against you.

Is this hard to do? And does it take a long time? It is a challenging process, yes, but very much worth it. And you will have moments of relapses, that is only to be expected, but read on because with the therapies I am going to show you, it will make the whole process that much easier.

Remember 'The Golden Rules'

O Drink hot water regularly with a slice of lemon in it to counteract the flight or fight response.

O Take Rescue Remedy every ten to fifteen minutes or so.

O Meditate once or twice daily.

◯ Eat some food (no stimulants with refined sugar).

◯ Sip regularly from a bottle of water with **Rescue Remedy** added. (8 drops) and any other **Bach** remedies you require.

◯ Take time out and sleep. Watch a **DVD** and switch off.

◯ Don't berate yourself for doing very little with your day. See it more looking after yourself and getting well again.

◯ See every slight improvement as a mile stone towards your wellbeing. And don't get disheartened if you have a bad day, it's just a bad day, tomorrow will be better.

◯ Talk with family or a trusted friend.

◯ Write down your worries.

◯ Take the mind set, the pain is just the anxiety leaving my body.

◯ Try not associating the pain with fear. The more fear you put into the sensations the more you feed the anxiety, resulting in stronger more frequent symptoms.

◯ Remember, you will come to no harm. 'YOU ARE SAFE.'

Summary

Tick

Box

☐ Almost in all cases, the symptoms you are feeling are a direct reaction to too much adrenaline in the body.

☐ Understanding why you are feeling such symptoms make

them less frightening.

☐Muscle tension is a good early warning system you are stressed.

☐Keep using the relaxation techniques, be kind on yourself.

☐Stop berating yourself, this has an immediate impact on your well being.

☐Structure your day, slow the rush rush rush.

☐Eat the right foods, (see chapter, *Diet and the Importance*' for further guidance).

☐Use the Bach flower remedies, e.g. *'Rescue Remedy.'*

☐Don't forget to praise yourself on all your achievements.

☐Allow the feelings and sensations to pass without paying any attention to them. By removing the fear you will gradually remove the symptoms.

☐'YOU ARE SAFE.'

- 8 -

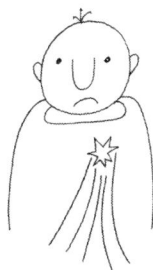

Emotions

Unplugged

Before we start the healing program, I'd just like to say opening up our emotions can be extremely painful, yet shouldn't be associated with any life threatening illness. Energy becomes blocked due to the stamping down of experiences, the ones we'd rather avoid and just forget about. But that's where illness can come. By not dealing with a particular emotion, shouting, screaming, crying, or confronting the pain, it becomes locked inside our bodies with no way of venting out. A wall becomes built as protection, and when confronted with a similar situation, we can't cope, instead we clamp down inside and wait for the situation to pass.

This is normal, we all want to avoid the bad bits in our lives and move forward, but when they aren't dealt with in the first place, that's where the problems can start. What we should do in an ideal world is deal with the problem(s) when they happen, then we wouldn't have the issue in the first place. But this doesn't come naturally, yet it is something you can learn, and be the better for it.

Recognising emotional blockages

Tick box

☐Have you tended to shy away from emotions?

☐Has somebody repeatedly told you not to cry because it's a weakness?

☐Do you feel afraid to show emotions?

☐Are you unsure what emotions you do feel?

☐Do you feel mixed and emotionally confused?

Again, these are all quite normal, but don't go beating yourself up over them. With time and patience things shall become clearer for you. But however much advice I can give, however high the amount of encouragement, the decision to get better has to come from you. You will need a strong desire to see this thing through to the end. To follow what I give you without giving in, otherwise the battle may be lost.

And remember. When you feel well in yourself once more, life will still create stress for you from time to time. Anxiety, or even panic might come back. Yet it's never too late to go back over this process and use the healing again. Every time you do this, the task will become slightly easier until it feels natural. But don't become angry or impatient if this happens, because with every episode, you'll become stronger inside, and you will never return to the person you were before. - Great strength will emerge.

Say, *'I get stronger every day in every way.'*

'Remember: Anxiety/Panic – feelings reduce with every attack conquered.'

In the positive, you will come out the other side with a greater understanding of yourself, what exactly makes you tick, and that life is there for living, not working every hour sent and collapsing tired and miserable. - You know, life should actually be fun; it's only other people who've told you it isn't. 'Only the lucky ones have a dream job' they say.

Well, actually no. It's a decision, nothing else.

The person made a decision, they wanted something and made it happen. What stops many of us is the fear. Think, how to make it happen, not, why it can't possibly work. Get excited. Your life can change. You don't have to put up with what you've got and be grateful for that. Go do what you want. Because panic can come if we feel trapped, stuck in a rut with no obvious way of getting out. But there is a way; you only have to begin by thinking it.

Six ways to combat emotional blockages

Bach flower remedies*

Crystal/Reiki/Spiritual healing*

Hypnotherapy*

Positive self talk*

Talking to somebody*

Keeping a diary*

---

*Discussed later in the book

Thought + Belief = Way forward

Things to remember when going through the healing process.

☐ Accept who we are.

☐ Treat ourselves as we would treat others.

☐ How can we love if we don't love ourselves first?

☐ Feed your body and your body will feed you.

☐ Rest is the best medicine.

☐ You are special, so believe it.

☐ Trust in the process of life, and life will trust in you.

☐ Smile, be happy. The higher your mood the better you feel.

☐ For today, do something that makes you feel happy.

☐ Listen to your heart and use your head, dreams are made here.

☐ Stick to your dreams, they make you.

☐ Believe in yourself and don't allow others to influence you.

☐ Live as you want to live, not how others think you should live.

☐ Take care and know you deserve better.

☐ Remember, you are safe.

Remedies to take: **Crab Apple,** for self acceptance and self love. **Rock Water,** not being so hard on yourself. **Walnut** for not being influenced by other people. Helps accept change.

- Section Two –

The Healing Programme

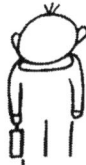

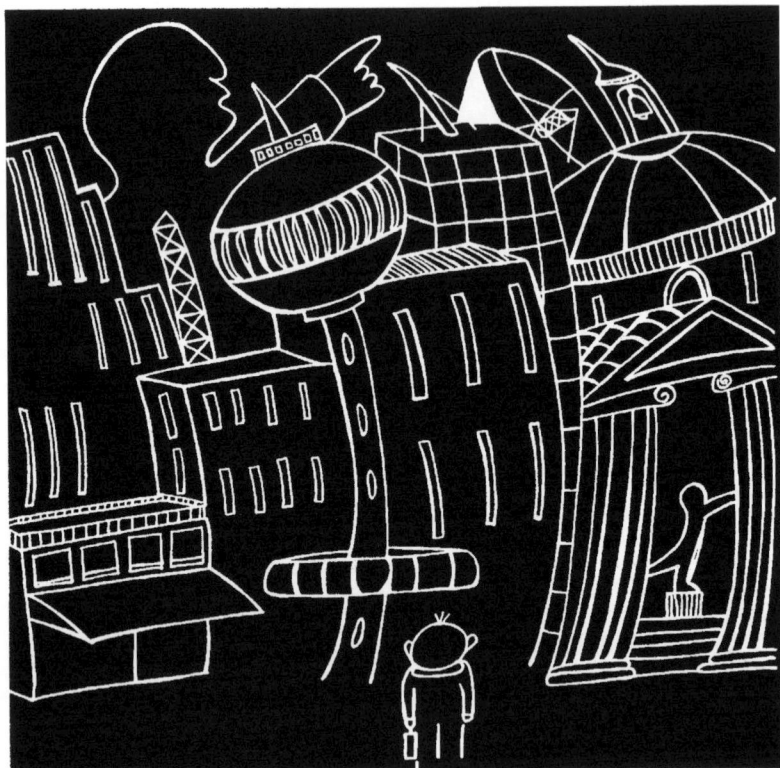

- 9 -

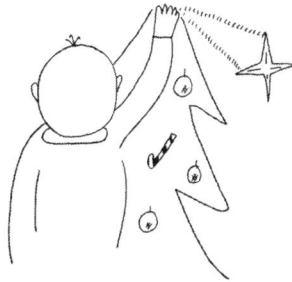

A Fallen Star

First step to Recovery

After trying many therapies and failing, I came to realise I was against a brick wall. I honestly thought I'd tried every avenue, but during the last moments of dying hope fate came to my rescue. Lady luck had waved her magic wand, and I soon found myself knocking on a stranger's door wondering whether the answer was the other side.

The time was early March 2003.

A hall light blinked on, and a man answered and let me in. I was shown into the sitting room where a group of woman and children sat busily chatting. I smiled. In truth it felt awkward. – Part of me demanded why I'd come. – While the other part wanted a cure. These were desperate times, and although I was in close proximity with people I'd never met, something kept saying stay. What did I have to lose?

Plucking some courage, I tried to make conversation with one of the ladies. But because how I felt at the time, it seemed strained. We didn't say very much to be truthful. She told me my energy was exiting out of the top of my head and needed capping fast. I looked at her wondering whether she was being serious, although by the lack of any expression evidently she was.

So there I sat not knowing what to expect. My early guess was a premixed bottle of Bach flower solution and out the door, with a thanks for coming, see you later type of approach. Yet as I was soon to discover this was not the case.

The stranger, Dawn, rushed past. She told me she wouldn't be long, and true to her word ten minutes later I was standing inside a nice purple room with angels and crystals all around. The room was calm; I felt quite nervous, overly self-conscious. Couldn't stop shaking but did my best to hide the fact. I wanted to look sane, I didn't want any more probing like the cognitive therapy had done, I just wanted a mixture that would take the panics away. I wanted sanity, I wanted someone to say, 'you're not going to die. You are safe.'

Dawn kindly showed me a seat.

This was a far cry from my previous endeavour, in front of me was someone who genuinely cared if I got better. A true warmth, a kindness so great I wasn't sure how to react at first. This was a genuine person. Someone who wouldn't say things behind your back, who'd be there for you when you fell into a dizzy crazed hole and needed a long lifeline to haul yourself out. - When that happened, rest assured, Dawn was at the other end smiling with hand outstretched. Which makes me think, if there are true angels who walk among us in our day to day lives, it's my conviction Dawn is one of them. Why else would someone help me?

I couldn't cope with life. I was twenty seven for Christ's sake, I jumped if there was a loud noise such as a phone, or car horn. What kind of person does that?

I can only guess she saw something worth saving, while I projected something completely different to what was going on inside. Yet Dawn wasn't fooled by outside appearances. She picked up my feelings from her natural intuition and knowledge to help with the remedy. - I didn't understand fully. But the thing which blew me away was how spot on she was. I felt like I'd walked in with a giant plaque spelling out what was wrong. – Someone actually knew. Jesus Christ, this was the turning point. The golden prize had come nearer.

As an extra, it never felt like we had to break the ice. We just got on. Conversation flowed easily, and soon enough, she'd done my remedies through the strength test, otherwise known as 'Kinesiology.' - But where Dawn was different to others, apart from her easy going positive manner, she showed an exceptional understanding in the human emotion department.

Not that I was wholly willing to let up all my problems in one sitting, some of them I didn't know, but with her guidance and remedies, I came to understand myself better. And I realised it's actually okay to ask for help, it's not a weakness. You don't have to bottle everything up and wait for the almighty explosion. Prevention can be achieved before total chaos comes near.

All too soon the first session ended and something unexpected happened. I stood by the front door searching for my keys when Dawn gave me a real big hug and told me to look after myself. I was surprised in the least. Not being used to hugs, especially from a near stranger, it threw me completely off track.

Keeping it together, I thanked her and walked out into the cool night with high expectations. I had a bottle of remedy in one hand, and a whole load of positive support behind me. – Support that I will cherish forever.

I will never forget what this gifted lady named Dawn did for me, how she turned a human stricken with deep fear, self hatred, and doubt, into somebody who could end up writing a book to help others in the same situation.

That night, things were beginning to look for the better, I was sure of that.

Over the following days I took the remedy and spoke to Dawn over the phone. The more we spoke a friendship grew, which I hope will never be lost. It was as though we were meant to meet, help each other through difficulties so our tarnished souls could shine a golden brilliance once more.

But if there is one thing I treasure, it's Dawn's trust. I feel honoured if I can help her in anyway, because if circumstances were different, and I'd never have met her, I know I'd be either stumbling in the wilderness, or encroaching upon suicide. Dawn believed in me. She said I should write and help others. I wanted this in the past, but having not found the answer, it would have surely failed. Timing was everything.

So when the time felt right, I started, and her encouragement has been immense. Never a put down or sarcastic remark, just pure kindness. I owe her my life.

I was all so happy on the outside, but inside, I was quietly dying in a slow tormenting pain. I had no control. I'd shake most of the time, felt dreadful, I didn't know whether I'd be alive from one minute to the next, and here was my beacon to follow. Dawn.

I guess I just wanted somebody to believe in me, was that really so much to ask?

Having somebody to pass dialogue with

Which leads me nicely to the next subject I'd like to discuss. - Talking.

We as humans need other humans to interact with; our nature makes us that way. And however withdrawn you feel, a sympathetic ear makes the world of difference.

It has to be someone you feel comfortable around, a person who generally cares, and is willing to listen and give positive constructive feedback. Not a person who tells you you're talking rubbish. Or ends up talking about themselves all the time. Because that is going to be of no use at all. On the other hand, there has to be give and take in the friendship. Listen to some of their worries as well, by doing this, it ensures the friendship shall last, instead of either party becoming bored and looking for answers someplace else. - You don't want bad feelings creating more of a problem than you originally started with.

Talking makes you realise you are not alone. You don't have to suffer in silence and internalise all the negatives, which tear you apart thus feeding the panic further. Simply by talking, it gets whatever's been thrashing about in your mind out in the open. And through discussion, problems will be resolved, other avenues you hadn't realised existed will make life more comfortable. It's powerful, and that's why I mention it here, just as with the act of writing down thoughts, (see next chapter) speaking them most certainly heals the soul.

Summary

Tick

Box

☐Find someone you can talk to.

☐It's okay to admit to somebody you need help.

☐Don't be nervous about talking about things. The more talking the greater the healing will happen for you.

☐You will need a connection with that person so you feel you can talk about anything in strict confidence.

☐Talking helps relieve negative thinking, while giving you reassurance everything is okay.

☐Use Bach flower remedy *'Agrimony'* to help you verbalise your emotions.

☐This is your first step towards recovery.

☐Remember, 'YOU ARE SAFE.'

- 10 -

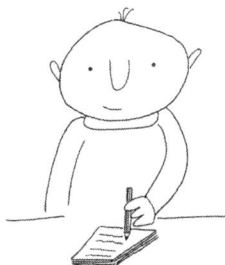

Keeping a Diary

Although finding a trusted somebody to talk with is powerful, it may not always be possible, or there are some things you might not want to talk about or feel you can. That's where a diary comes in.

A diary can help in a couple of ways:

1. Recognising a panic attack is coming on so you can deal with it.

2. Handle day to day destructive thoughts which lead to feeling unwell.

When an attack is building, it's not always easy to remember the tell tale signs. You might think it's all just down to tiredness because you've been working hard as late. That might be true, exhaustion brings symptoms, but if these symptoms appear regularly, and just before an attack, some kind of record will be advantageous for warning them off.

You'll see them coming and act accordingly, diminishing their strength or putting off the whole episode altogether. Great! I hear you cry, that's that solved. And yes, in a way it is. But like all methods, you'll need to practice until the message filters through, and the release trigger becomes desensitised.

That's part of it, but we have something more destructive to deal with here. As mentioned before, and as you will soon discover through a coming chapter, your past problems have a strong hold on the way you act and cope today. We need to know the past and break it. We also need to know what's churning today, tomorrow and the next day. There might be some new ones that seemingly pop up out of nowhere, but with some careful deduction, they'll most likely harp back to your past again. Something which had a dramatic influence on you back then.

And now, when you're put in a certain situation? It suddenly all becomes very difficult to cope again. Fortunately we can start to readdress negative thinking through the act of writing it down.

'Replace the negative thoughts with positive ones until they become your reality.'

(Dawn Chrystal 2004)

So this is your first task. Find yourself a diary, or use your computer, tablet, or mobile phone. Whatever works for you and you can access easily. Now write. Write whatever comes into your mind. However crazy you might think these thoughts are, write them down, however destructive, write them down. This is your new healing ground; this is where things will get better because you have now started to offload your worries and air them. Something that can be hard to do at first, even upsetting, but will be well worth it in the long run. - Write every day. Don't let up. Make this a new habit.

Now, this is the part where we take the negatives from your diary and turn them into positives. Glance through what you have written and take a fresh piece of paper. Write down the first negative you see and underneath write a positive counteraction. Good. Now write out the positive three times and read only the positive several times over to get it in your head. Do this negative positive exercise for everything you have written, e.g.

The negative – positive diary

Today's date: 16/3/04

Negative: I felt awful today, why won't these pains go away??

Positive: I know this process is gradual I am working through it. I am getting stronger.

Positive: I know this process is gradual I am working through it. I am getting stronger.

Positive: I know this process is gradual I am working through it. I am getting stronger.

Negative: I needed to work but all I could think of was if this is the end for me.

Positive: I managed to get through work today I can do the same tomorrow.

Positive: I managed to get through work today I can do the same tomorrow.

Positive: I managed to get through work today I can do the same tomorrow.

Say: *'Everyday in every way I am getting stronger and stronger.'*

Also repeat to yourself: *'Panic is not my reality anymore.'*

See how it works? – For each day you write down all the negatives, this acts as a clearing process, and below, you write about the positives. However small they might be, jot them down. Anything is better than nothing. It will be the positives you shall be concentrating on from today onwards. They will give you your strengths.

And once you've finished filling in all your negatives and positives, take a pair of scissors and cut away the negatives. Keep the positive side somewhere safe, in a box file, or a paper folder. But where the negative are concerned, they can be torn up, burnt, or also placed in a file. Only the negative should never see the light of day again.

The reason being, it may hurt you. It can churn you inside, push you deeper in that dark hole and bring on the pains. Believe me, this should not be taken lightly. The power of the word should not be underestimated. Because when you read the past negatives, it's kicking off memories, the type of memories which fool your brain into thinking it's happening all over again. And for obvious reasons, you don't want that.

On the other hand, by re-reading your positives, it has the opposite effect. It lifts your mood, you can see progress is being made, and all your hard efforts are gradually bearing fruit. It shows you there is light at the end of the tunnel.

'When the mind's ranting about something or other, and all you want is to settle down and forget it, the diary has the power to do that. It can also bring positive thought, which counteracts the way you are feeling with the panics.'

Summary

Tick

Box

☐A diary helps you understand the warning signals of an impending panic attack, this allows you to recognise and prevent before it's too late.

☐A diary is a simple way of moving negative thoughts to a place they can't harm.

☐Refrain from reading over the negative you've written, it can bring back past negatives which are destructive to feeling better and moving forward.

☐Re-read all the positives for each day, they will prove you are making progress while cancelling out all the harmful negative thoughts.

☐Your diary represents your own personal thoughts, keep it secret, or only show the most trusted of friends.

☐Write every day, make it a new habit.

☐'YOU ARE SAFE.'

- 11 -

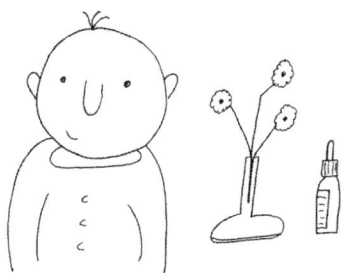

Bach Flower Remedies

Heal your mind and your body will follow

Remember when you opened this book and I instructed you to get hold of some *'Rescue Remedy'*, and obtain yourself some strength through relaxation, before continuing on your journey in the quest of good health?

And you did it didn't you. – Because why would you buy a self help book and leave it on the side to gather dust, especially without trying the methods detailed within? – It wouldn't make any sense.

So having done this, a feeling of calmer waters are upon you. You believed in the remedy, you were willing for change, and now you can start to feel a difference. It might be small. A slight reduction in overall anxiety levels, a cut in the severity or number of attacks. But nevertheless, progress has come, and you are beginning to understand the importance of taking Bach flower remedies.

With that firmly locked in your mind, I want you to use a Bach flower practitioner and have the remedies mixed to your particular state of mind. Whether it's depression, lack of go, fear, impatience, stuck in the past, or whatever. This little bottled miracle sent from Mother Nature, courtesy of Mr. Bach, is waiting for you.

Take it in hand. Embrace this chance of getting better. - Yes you're feeling battered and bruised, that's understandable, you've been through a heck of a lot recently. And then there's the strong fear of toppling over insanity's edge to deal with. But you're okay, really you are. You've managed the first major steps into recovery. And although every cell in that body of yours is screaming out for rest, you're not going to lie down and give up on me. You're going to say, back off panic attacks, I'm going to the next stage, which is really going to kick some butt. In fact, Mr. Anxiety, you're going to regret ever picking on me in the first place.

What comes with a strong mind is control. With control, comes a new era for you. A time in the not too distant future where you'll sit back and relax, feeling proud of what you've achieved here. The battle shall be won.

Now use that little bit of confidence to good effect by gauging what you're actually dealing with here. Go make it your big mission to seek someone genuine who deals in these wonderful remedies. It won't take long to find someone, there are many people out there, just be careful who you ultimately choose. Chat to them for a while, gauge their enthusiasm for the subject, which is always a good indication you're on the right track. You know the signs, the eyes that twinkle, the distant look, a smile matched with a choice of words that can only come when someone is deeply passionate in their vocation. When you see this, make an appointment and keep regular meetings, making sure your remedies are adjusted to present state of feelings. Normally every two weeks, but can often be shorter the closer you are to the finishing line.

For me. I found Dawn. My saviour from what I'm sure was verging on madness. Her acute ability to read a person's emotions, advice on life changing methods such as positive self talk, and looking to the future instead of the past, coaxed me out of the dark hole we sufferers know all too well about. I was shown the way towards a brighter light, where I could start to grow as a person again, instead of running and hiding like my past patterns had led me to.

But a quick word of warning. Don't be attracted by those who charge the earth for a quick fix. Find someone like Dawn, who genuinely cares in making you better and the future look brighter. Follow their guidance, and never doubt great strength will emerge from within.

How does it work?

The practitioner will mix a bottle to the precise feelings you're battling with at that moment. A good healer shall be able to sense your mood and mix accordingly over the phone. Face to face, they'll adopt a different method, testing your strength against the remedy bottle.

It works on your subconscious. By holding one of the 38 bottles to your cheek, your healer shall ask you to hold your other arm out straight. By pushing down on that arm, the subconscious decides whether you need that particular remedy or not. A weak arm indicates yes, where a strong arm is no. A further 37 bottles later, you'll have your mixture, accompanied with the positive and negative for each.

For an example, look at the following:

Rock Rose

Negative state – Acute fears, terror & panic.

Positive state – Great courage – Is willing to risk life for others. Self is forgotten. Strength of will and character.

It might not always immediately become obvious when explained, but with some thinking, you'll begin to recognise why the remedy has come up, giving you a better understanding of why you feel the way you do. Don't dismiss it straightaway, that's just denying yourself from getting to the bottom of this. You have to want to find out, and break down the barriers that have made you the way you are. Think of it like a demolition job. Okay you might know nothing about blowing up buildings, but in your imagination, who cares?

Exercise: - *'Picture yourself inserting dynamite into the wall you're fighting. Imagine the word relevant to you, such as PANIC, in large letters on that wall. Now watch what happens when you stand back and push that huge red plunger down. See the violent explosion as big and as loud as you can, and when the dust has finally settled, walk forward ready to tackle the next problem.'*

In my view, Bach flower remedies are an essential tool when overcoming panic. They not only help you understand yourself better, but they gently turn your negative patterns into positive. Which is why without them it would make the task much harder than needs be.

'Flower remedies help us gently peel back our negative emotions so we can deal with them and release them fully.'

Listening in on a session

I now want you to pretend you're doing a bit of eaves dropping. You're standing at the door listening to Dawn carrying out the remedy test on myself. This will help you understand what's entailed, and how easy it will be for you to undertake.

Dawn's just completed the muscle test and has the bottles in front of her on a table. 'I can see you are suffering from feeling guilty,' she says, 'therefore we have **Pine** here. This will help with *self respect.'*

I nod, not quite believing such a simple method has pinpointed what I'm feeling.

Dawn puts her finger on the second bottle. 'Next there's a feeling of not liking oneself, so **Crab Apple** for starting to *accept and like yourself.'*

'I see that,' I say, feeling a bit tearful. Yet trying desperately not to embarrass myself.

Dawn turns another bottle round to disclose the label. *'Cerato. Self doubt with loss of identity.* This will help with *trusting yourself.'*

Another big one for me. People would say what a fine job I'd done at work, but I couldn't see it. I never trusted in myself that I had done a good job.

'Star of Bethlehem for *shocks and trauma's.* This will help you deal with them more easily.'

I wasn't surprised by this one. The attacks themselves had left a lot of this behind. Not to mention what my self destructive thoughts were doing.

Dawn picks up a bottle with **Rock Water** on the front. 'For *being too hard on yourself.* You need to lighten up. Beating yourself is just making the problem worse.'

Again I could see that. But I didn't think I was good enough, I didn't like myself. I hated being me.

'Extreme mental anguish and reaching limit of endurance. For this I give you **Sweet Chestnut.** It shall quiet that mind of yours and help you see the light at the end of the tunnel.'

My mind was racing all the time with negative thoughts. If it wasn't about myself, it was about me dying, I couldn't concentrate on anything else.

'And here we have **Rock Rose**, this will help *calm the panics.'*

I wanted the whole bottle, not just a few drops. If there was one remedy I needed more than the others, this was it. To get rid of the feelings of panic.

Dawn gazes over the other bottles. 'There are others that have shown up,' she says, 'but for the moment, I'm rather declined in giving them to you right now. Not until you feel stronger. We don't want the whole process to bring you down further than need be.'

I put a couple of drops on my tongue while she continues.

'It's worth mentioning, the causes for panic attacks are quite often not what we expect. *Emotions, such as anger or low self esteem, are trigger points.'*

I wasn't so sure. All I could feel was fear, and that was bubbling up inside me so much I hurt all over. But I put my trust in what Dawn was saying, because she knew, she'd seen it all before in herself and others, so I wasn't going to try and dispute the fact. I just wanted the panic to go away so I could feel better.

Next Dawn shows me the positives and how important it is to concentrate on them. I promised to keep this up, which I think pleased her. There is nothing as infuriating as trying to help somebody who doesn't want to change. But I did, and the second session in two weeks would be interesting.

'To summarise, my mix of flower remedies were not uncommon for a panic attack sufferer. In fact, Dawn finds these come up nearly every time with new clients with this problem.'

Pine – Self respect.

Crab Apple – To accept and like yourself.

Cerato – For trusting your own gut instinct.

Star of Bethlehem – Softens shocks and trauma's.

Rock Water – For being gentler on yourself.

Sweet Chestnut – For seeing light at the end of the tunnel. Your prayers shall be answered.

Rock Rose – Calm the panics.

14 days later, and I started to see the changes. Dawn explained the feelings I felt were quite normal. Bach remedies are a gentle way of easing you from the gloomy outlook you had on life, into the positive. By doing this, I became stronger, I found myself dealing with situations I'd otherwise would have run from.

My brother's wedding for example. I was dreading the day. Seeing family members I felt awkward around, strangers staring, dancing. Making small talk. Enough to make the sanest of us worried. Yet with Dawn's guidance, I flew through the event, and nothing became a problem because I didn't let it. The strength the remedies gave me allowed a platform for confidence to grow from. - And where I once cared what strangers thought of me, now I couldn't care less. That's the miracle. Use with positive self talk, and the moon's a doddle. Heck, even mars looks realistic from here.

So where had I gone wrong? I was digging myself into a deeper hole; I was horrible. - To me! The one person I should be especially nice too. But no. I had decided to beat myself up, and now it all becomes clear.

I was feeling ill because of my thoughts, how I perceived others to see me. My programming had been messed up by those who I'd come into contact with, and now I'd manifested into my worst enemy. You get used to this, you do it without realising, you react to situations that caused trauma in the past but wonder why you feel the way you do. But suddenly, as you start to feel stronger, and the more positive you feel about yourself, the more everything makes sense. You'll start to change and feel better for it. However, berate yourself, and all too easily that chest pain comes back, making you realise what you've slipped back into. – Time to now change the pattern, the remedy helps you to do so.

Bach flower directory

To finish this chapter off, I'm going to introduce you to the Bach Flower Directory which lists the full 38 bottles. This will help identify your emotion easily with the corresponding remedy to use for rectification. I've included this, so if you do initially fancy having a go yourself, you'll be able to self diagnose and mix your own bottle. Highly useful if you find yourself going downwards with a known reason, you'll be able to get back on track without having to make an appointment with your practitioner.

A few pointers:

○ Don't underestimate the power of talking, and having someone's help in recognising how you feel.

○ Self diagnosis's is o.k., but your practitioner will become invaluable in aiding your recovery. Especially when working through past problems and putting everything back in perspective.

○ There are 38 flower remedies which all have a specific purpose.

○ Each remedy has the power to turn negative into positive.

○ Although your feelings may become heightened for a short period, relax, they will pass, leaving you with a more positive outlook on life.

○ Remember to take your remedy regularly.

○ Drink plenty of water.

○ 'YOU ARE SAFE.'

Directory

Remedy - Agrimony

Negative - Puts on a brave face to hide problems. Avoid confrontation.

Positive outcome - Ability to confront and verbalise emotions.

Remedy - Aspen

Negative - Unexplained fears and worries. Nervous and anxious.

Positive outcome - Overcome and trust.

Remedy - Beech

Negative - Critical and intolerant of others. Judgmental and fault finding.

Positive outcome - Tolerance and understanding

Remedy – Centuary

Negative - Has difficulty in saying no. Anxious to please. Easily influenced.

Positive outcome - Strength to stand up for oneself. Ability to say 'NO!'

Remedy - Cerato

Negative - Doubts own ability and intuition. Loss of identity.

Positive outcome - Inner certainty & self assurance.

Remedy - Cherry Plum

Negative - Fear of losing mind. P.M.T. Irrational thoughts or behaviour.

Positive outcome - Mental calm.

Remedy - Chestnut Bud

Negative - Fails to learn from experience. Repeats same mistakes.

Positive outcome - Learns from mistakes so doesn't repeat them.

Remedy - Chicory

Negative - Overly possessive, expects others to conform. Enjoys an argument.

Positive outcome - Brings care and love for others.

Remedy - Clematis

Negative - Daydreams, lack of interest in present.

Positive outcome - Centres, creates contact with reality and present.

Remedy - Crab Apple

Negative - Poor self image, ashamed or embarrassed by physical symptoms, characteristics or features. Lack of self love.

Positive outcome - Cleanses the system. Acceptance of self.

Remedy - Elm

Negative - Overwhelmed or burdened by responsibility and exhaustion.

Positive outcome - Relief from feeling heavy load.

New self assurance.

Remedy -Gentian

Negative - Easily discouraged, hesitant and despondent. Pessimistic.

Positive outcome - Optimism faith and encouragement.

Remedy - Gorse

Negative - Feels hopelessness and despair, pessimistic. Dark under eyes, ashen faced.

Positive outcome - Renewed faith and hope. Good start to speedy recovery.

Remedy - Heather

Negative - Feel self-absorbed, dislike being alone, are excessively talkative.

Positive outcome - Creates empathy and a readiness to help others.

Remedy - Holly

Negative - Feelings of extreme jealousy, envy and suspicion. Anger.

Positive outcome - Brings feelings of love and tolerance.

Remedy - Honeysuckle

Negative - Lives in the past, homesick or nostalgic.

Positive outcome - Lays past to rest and moves forward.

Remedy - Hornbeam

Negative - Monday morning feeling. Unable to face the day. Procrastination.

Positive outcome - Creates vitality, strengthens mind.

Remedy - Impatiens

Negative - Impatient, easily irritated. Short temper.

Positive outcome - Encourages gentleness and patience.

Remedy - Larch

Negative - Lack of self confidence, feelings of being inferior. Expects failure.

Positive outcome - Feelings of confidence.

Remedy - Mimulus

Negative - Has a fear rooted in known cause.

Positive outcome - Gives courage. Strength and understanding.

Remedy - Mustard

Negative - Deep gloom which comes and goes for no apparent reason, can be caused by unrecognised anger.

Positive outcome - Gives clarity and happiness.

Remedy - Oak

Negative - Driven by a strong sense of duty and struggles on though exhausted.

Positive outcome - Strength and endurance.

Remedy - Olive

Negative - Exhausted in mind and body.

Positive outcome – Revitalises.

Remedy - Pine

Negative - Guilt, blame self for others mistakes. Not honouring own needs.

Positive outcome - Relieves guilt, encourage feelings of forgiveness of self.

Remedy - Red Chestnut

Negative - Over anxious or over-concern for others.

Positive outcome - Positive thinking and ability to remain calm. Radiates positive to others. Good for carers.

Remedy - Rescue Remedy

Negative – Used in demanding or stressful situations.

Positive outcome - Good initial remedy for panic attacks.

Remedy - Rock Rose

Negative - Experience of terror, been frozen in fear and helplessness.

Positive outcome - Courage and calm.

Remedy - Rock Water

Negative - Inflexible, sets very high standards for themselves.

Positive outcome - Adaptability, open mind. Kinder to self.

Remedy - Scleranthus

Negative - Indecision, fluctuating moods, loss of balance.

Positive outcome - Balance and determination.

Remedy - Star of Bethlehem

Negative - Experienced shock, grief, or fright.

Positive outcome - Comforts and soothes.

Remedy - Sweet Chestnut

Negative - Limits of endurance, deep despair. Isolation. Desire to hide from the world.

Positive outcome - Releases anxiety. Light at the end of the tunnel.

Continued...

Remedy - Vervain

Negative - Over-enthusiastic. Argumentative with fixed principles and ideas.

Positive outcome - Relaxation, self discipline.

Remedy - Vine

Negative - Strong willed, domineering or inflexible. Wants control and can be quite ruthless.

Positive outcome - Positive leadership and inspiration.

Remedy - Walnut

Negative - Facing major life changes, need protection from influences of others, over sensitivity.

Positive outcome - Helps adapt to change, protects from others influences.

Remedy - Water Violet

Negative - Prefers to be alone. Isolated. Too proud to ask for help.

Positive outcome - Share and socialize. Quite gentle and sympathetic.

Remedy - White Chestnut

Negative - Have unwanted thoughts, preoccupied and worried. Sleeplessness and frontal headaches.

Positive outcome - Calm and peace of mind. Controlled thoughts.

Remedy - *Wild Oat*

Negative - Frustration and dissatisfaction with lifestyle, uncertain which path to follow.

Positive outcome - Assists in purpose of life.

Remedy - *Wild Rose*

Negative - Makes little effort to improve situation. Lack of interest or motivation. Boredom and tiredness.

Positive - Helps regain enthusiasm for life. Ambitious and purposeful.

Remedy - *Willow*

Negative - Resentful and have feelings of self pity.

Positive outcome - Optimism and faith.

Buy flower remedies online, visit website:

www.creaturecomforters.co.uk

I personally use Creature Comforters for my flower remedies, aura and energy sprays, because of their very high quality and professional service.

Note: As Rescue Remedy is a proprietary name, it also comes under the names *'Five Flower Essence,'* *'Emergency Essence,'* and *'Comforter'* etc.

Summary

Tick

Box

☐Find a good Bach remedy practitioner, and have the remedies tailor made for maximum effect.

☐Bach remedies hold the power for positive change.

☐You can utilise the directory at the end of this chapter for self diagnosis.

☐Self diagnosis is o.k. But remember, your therapist will be of great help in your recovery.

☐Bach remedies can be used with any existing medication you may be on, though you may wish to consult your doctor beforehand.

☐Bach remedies are a natural healer, but should not be regarded as a replacement to prescribed medicine if they are appropriate.

☐Remember, **'YOU ARE SAFE'**

-12-

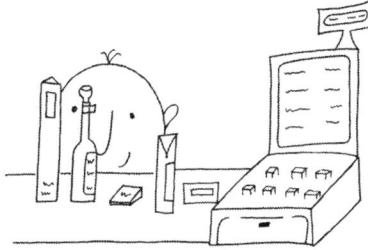

Diet and the Importance

Maybe once or twice a week, depending on the type of car you drive, you fill up your tank with fuel and you know you're set for roughly a certain number of miles. That makes sense, without fuel, you're going nowhere. You might as well be sitting in a garden shed, because the car won't turn a wheel without the gasoline to propel it. - Exactly the same goes for you.

You might be thinking, I'm okay, I eat well enough. But are you? Are you really fuelling up as needed, or are you half starving your body of what it really requires?

It's a tough one to answer for sure, especially when dealing with panic attacks, because much of the time food seems like the last thing on your mind. The sick feelings won't go away, so you tend to starve and only eat when you feel better. For the simple fact, your body is preparing itself to flee. It wants to lighten itself so you can travel faster. It just doesn't realise this is an inappropriate time for your fight or flight response to be kicking in.

So what can you do? How can you overcome this and eat appropriately?

A little of what you like is a good starting point. Find some food that you loved before all this started, and you know won't have any adverse effects.

For me, it was those readymade pancakes with raisins and some melted butter on top. The slow release energy of the raisins helped me enormously, yet was gentle enough not to cramp my stomach and have me rushing for the nearest toilet.

Why slow release? Slow release sustains an even amount of energy instead of short rapid bursts like caffeine and chocolate produce. By maintaining this, *'even energy level,'* the body doesn't tip into the extreme, making everything run much faster than you want it too.- You have to remember, your body has a lot of adrenaline pumping around through anxiety, so adding more energy, only makes the symptoms worse. Then you worry what's happening to you, more adrenaline is put into the system, you feel worse, and so on. The cycle goes round again – Of course you'll get to a point you can't feel any worse, but why make everything so bad? Especially when all you have to do is watch what you're putting inside yourself. And at the end of the day, prevention is better than cure.

'Slow release foods – Try healthy cereal bars instead of chocolate, and perhaps a tub of raisins. Use them to supplement your daily intake. – Also rye, oats, and barley are good slow release foods.'

By helping the body feel better, strength wise, this has an added advantage of knocking on to your mental state.

For example. When everything was calm inside, did you continually think about an attack coming on? Was there any deep dread inside, wondering whether the awful might happen &

you'd be in a state of panic before the day was out?

The answer, probably not. That's because our minds are great forgetters where pain is concerned. We don't tend to dwell on pain when we feel good and happy within ourselves, which is a saving grace. But constantly running back over old ground shocks the body, and can bring the symptoms all over again.

So it's fair to say, our diet can have an enormous influence on our well being where the energy aspect is concerned. We are after all energy forms; as much as we are affected by stress and emotional baggage, the wrong food can have a detrimental effect on our well being. The right food is healing on mind and body.

Remember:

Negative Food in = Negative Output

Positive Food in = Positive Output

Foods to avoid

In the beginning, I said avoid caffeine for very good reasons. Technically, caffeine is a substance extracted from plants, or produced synthetically, for use as an additive in certain food products. It is a stimulant to the central nervous system and acts as a diuretic. You'll find it naturally in the leaves, seeds and fruit of more than sixty plants. Other than the obvious like coffee, caffeine can be found in tea, chocolate, cocoa, and many fizzy drinks. Not to mention, medications such as pain relievers, appetite suppressants, and cold medicines.

To give you an idea, a normal cup of coffee can have up to one hundred milligrams of caffeine, which is enough to notice significant effects on the body within thirty minutes of drinking. That's taking into account your average Joe with no health issues whatsoever, throw in anxiety, and now you're looking at a whole different issue.

The bottom line? Caffeine increases blood pressure, metabolic rate, and heart rate. Not to mention nervousness, irritability, and difficulty sleeping. Which is why, when you are suffering from an increased state of panic, taking caffeine in one form or another takes you onto the next stage of elevation. It can be something simple like a single piece of chocolate, or a sweet, but the outcome is as follows:

○ Pounding heart.

○ Nausea.

○ Vomiting.

○ Insomnia.

○ Shaking.

○ Ringing ears.

○ Sweaty palms.

Increase the intake of caffeine, and the symptoms heighten, but the real danger lies when you begin to feel these symptoms and misread them as something more serious.

The obvious answer would be to avoid caffeine altogether, but if it's already too late, drink plenty of water and control the breathing. The breathing will calm you down, while the water will weaken the caffeine and bring the symptoms back under control. It works relatively fast, yet reminds you to stay off the caffeine in the future.

And if some of the nice things in life have just been cruelly eradicated from your palette's desire, no fear, there are plenty of other foods to be discovered that will take their place.

Avoid:

O Processed foods and foods that create stress on the system. e.g.

O Artificial sweeteners.

O Chocolate.

O Eggs.

O Fried foods.

O Junk foods.

O Pork & red meat. (If you can't do without meat, try cutting down on the intake).

O Refined sugar.

O White flour products.

O Foods which contain preservatives or heavy spices.

O Chips & similar snack foods.

O Cheap oil. (Use olive oil in spray form).

Breakfast is for wimps!

Remember Del boy in the hit T.V. comedy 'Only fools and horses?' His line was such. But without breakfast, he became tired, couldn't think so clearly, and not to mention very very hungry.

Breakfast is our first fuel stop of the day after an average of eight hours sleep, the body needs this fuel to start functioning properly, so it's not surprising it's vital we fuel up accordingly. But it shouldn't be too heavy. You don't want to be suffering indigestion on the way to work; but fruit, fruit juice, and cereals are an excellent source for breakfast.

○ On waking, have a glass of warm water with a slice of lemon/lime to flush the system. This removes any excess acid and old food particles that may still be in the stomach from the day before. - Also aids bowel movements.

○ You can also use this to calm an unsettled stomach.

Things to remember for breakfast time

○ Try getting up early to give you plenty of time.

○ Perhaps prepare your breakfast things the night before.

○ Try not to rush your mornings.

○ Eat slowly, read the paper, talk.

○ Try not to allow your mind to become over busy with the days tasks. Write a list and concentrate on one job at a time.

○ Don't rush out the moment you finish, relax, ten minutes will make a large difference to your day.

○ Breakfast is the most important meal of the day, enjoy it.

○ Eating good healthy food gives positive results for the mind and body.

○ Food has the ability to help you heal naturally.

Say, 'today, I am in control of everything I do.'

Say, 'nothing will get in my way.'

'I can do this, and, I am safe.'

Breakfast and the rest of the day

The ideal breakfast foods are: grapes, apples, pears, papaya. **(Simple carbohydrates).**

Also: Cereal or porridge. **(Complex carbohydrates).**

Rye biscuits or rice cakes. **(Complex carbohydrates).**

Milk or soya milk. **(Protein).**

Cottage cheese or yogurt. **(Protein).**

Delay having a hot drink for at least fifteen to twenty minutes after. If you've eaten yogurt, wait until a couple of hours after breakfast, because it's not good for the bacteria.

A good breakfast based on proteins and complex carbohydrates will give the body enough energy for the mornings work.

Break time

Break times are often missed, or a cup of something is quickly gulped while on the move. This has the effect of stressing the body and making us feel unwell. Just five minutes rest every so often calms the system, and makes a dramatic difference on overall stress levels.

Some pointers:

O **Keep off the coffee and chocolate.**

O Stay away from sugary snacks.

O Have very weak tea, herbal, or plain water with a slice of lemon and lime.

O Concentrate on resting.

Lunch

By lunch time your body is asking for more fuel. For most of us, this is usually a quick sandwich from the local shop, but although this might be ideal for our lifestyle, it's not exactly ideal for our body.

Things to lunch on:

O Washed salad.

O Jacket potato with a topping. Like; tuna, cheese. (Try goats cheese, especially if you have a dairy intolerance).

O Ready cooked chicken pieces in a wrap with salad.

O Tuna sandwich with low fat mayonnaise.

O Fresh or dried fruit.

All these are readily available from either your local shop or supermarket. Not to mention many sandwich shops, who are now branching out into this field as well.

Again, take time to eat and don't rush your food. The digestive system needs you to be rested instead of diverting energies elsewhere.

Dinner

Because by now you've eaten a good breakfast backed up with a lunch of healthy proportions, dinner doesn't have to be a heavy affair. This is the time to unwind from the day's stresses and strains and sit down to enjoy what's on your plate. Forget what's been troubling you and relax. Talk, laugh, make this more of an occasion rather than a quick dash because you want to get somewhere. – In fact, give yourself enough time and you'll feel as though you can do something in the evening, rather than feeling overly tired and wanting just to sleep. Which might currently be a frustration for you. You want to do such and such but you don't have the energy. Well maybe now you do.

Recommended foods

Apricots, asparagus, avocados, bananas, broccoli, brown rice, dried fruits, figs, fish (notably salmon), garlic, green leafy vegetables, legumes, raw nuts, seeds, brewer's yeast, whole grains, soy products, and yogurt. These foods supply valuable minerals such as calcium, magnesium, phosphorus, and potassium, which are all depleted by stress.

'Eat a diet of 50 to 75 percent raw foods. Fresh fruit and vegetables supply valuable vitamins and minerals.'

Multivitamins

Multivitamins can be extremely beneficial when dealing with panic attacks. The body uses up certain vitamins and minerals when under stress, and obviously they need to be replaced. (See next page on these).

And food would normally do this, but food is grown for the mass market and at the greatest possible speed, and because of this, the food has a much depleted nutrient content than it did a hundred years ago.

So, for example sake, to get the same vitamin C from one orange, then, you'd actually have to eat between eight and ten each day!

And that's just not practical; nobody can consume those kinds of numbers in a single day, which is why multivitamins are becoming more important than they have been in the past.

By supplementing your daily food, you are at least getting some of the vitamins and minerals you require to keep your body healthy and working as it should.

But I have to say, I felt much better by taking a standard vitamin supplement. The type you find at your local supermarket costing not much more than a pound. And although for little cost, I felt stronger inside, less sick, and the anxiety level was that much lower. – These are my personal findings, yet you must decide for yourself whether to take supplements or not. Which is why, it might be a good idea to ask your doctor first, and maybe have an appointment with a nutritionist for total peace of mind.

Advantages of supplements commonly present in off the shelf multivitamins & mineral tablets

Supplement – Comments

Calcium

A natural tranquilizer.

Magnesium

Helps relieve anxiety tension, nervousness, and muscular spasms. Best taken with calcium.

Iron

Iron deficiency can increase the risk of panic attacks.

B12

Helps reduce stress and anxiety.

Potassium

Essential for proper functioning of the adrenal glands.

Selenium

A powerful anti-oxidant that protects the heart.

Also lifts moods and decreases anxiety.

B1 (Thiamine)

Reduces anxiety and calms the nerves.

Vitamin B6

A known energizer that exerts calm.

Vitamin C

Necessary for the proper function of the adrenal glands and brain chemistry. This is known to reduce anxiety due to its tranquilizing properties.

Vital when dealing with stress.

Vitamin E

Helps transport oxygen to brain cells and protects them from free radical damage.

Zinc

Calms the central nervous system.

Chromium

Chromium deficiency can produce symptoms of anxiety. This is most notable in people who consume large volumes of refined sugar.

Vitamin B Complex

All vitamin B's are necessary for good health and correct functioning of the nervous system.

'Try, Omega 3 (Fish oil) capsules. For efficient functioning of the nerves, helps protect the heart. And Theanine – An amino acid found in green tea known for its calming effects. – Luckily both are available in tablet form for ease.'

Also:

Fennel relieves anxiety-related gastrointestinal upsets. Good for reducing abdominal tension, wind, and relaxing the large intestine. Most effective when taken as a tea. Take before or after meals. Has no known side effect.

Also try Lemon balm and willow bark.

Peppermint tea calms the buildup of acid in the stomach. The acid is due to increased adrenaline through stress. - Peppermint is also available in capsules.

Skullcap and valerian root can be used at bedtime to aid sleep and help prevent panic attacks in the night.

I.B.S

Which brings me to the foods which might cause more discomfort as a sufferer of I.B.S, or Irritable Bowel Syndrome. You might never have heard of this, but there's a strong possibility you were a sufferer way before the attacks came on. Signs can be:

Physical: Bloating of the stomach after eating. Stomach cramps, heartburn, shaking, wind, and sickness. The need to repeatedly go to the toilet.

Mental: Find it difficult to cope in a new place associated with different people and not knowing where the nearest toilet is. Feel dirty and embarrassed by the condition, and would rather not enter a situation if there's a chance a cramp will strike.

Why some people suffer and others don't, isn't fully understood, but stress can certainly heighten the problem. But if you do suffer, and have found it difficult to cope with, you'll be pleased to know there is help at hand. You can make things easier through an exercise of detection and omission.

The elimination table

Food/Drink	Result	Toleration - 0-5
Banana	No effect	5
Curry	Big effect	0

By filling out this simple elimination table every time you eat, you will begin to understand what foods to stay away from, and which are safe. It might look laborious at first hand, but after a couple of weeks, you'll be surprised how much of an understanding you will have gained over the types of food and drink you'd do best to avoid. And by doing this, your stomach will stay calmer, energies will improve, and you'll feel a certain zest for life you once thought might never return. Not to mention the confidence factor, where you'll be able to deal with life's ups and downs that bit better. Like knowing you can get on that train without any repercussions, or stay in that important meeting without having to dash out half way through for the toilet. Again, it's a mind game.

Looking back at the *'Elimination table,'* I have included a toleration number which you can mark out of five. 0 is never again, five is normal. The reason being, you might find some foods are acceptable in small doses, but if you pig out, disaster occurs. Obviously after a while you'll be able to discard the chart, but for the moment, just keep it with you until you get a handle on this.

Intolerances

Gluten /wheat free and dairy free

This is something I wanted to add for a number of reasons. A couple of years back I was getting bouts of distressing stomach cramps, shaking, and the most painful indigestion that only fuelled my faulty belief system there was indeed something physically wrong with me. And this is an easy trap to fall into. It's hard enough to cope with anxiety alone, but this added extra burden, can not only make the symptoms worse, but fuel more fear which leads to faulty health anxiety thinking. So my advice is, try not to worry if you find yourself in the same situation, instead, do what I did, look for the answers by reading up and changing your diet. Intolerances can be confusing, painful, and debilitating. Everything you eat seems to be making you ill, and you feel so scared of eating you give up. But again, don't worry, there is a solution.

Gluten intolerance

Gluten intolerance does seem to be on the increase, and although it doesn't directly create anxiety, it does cause symptoms that will worry and affect the anxiety you are feeling. It is very uncomfortable and best dealt with by changing your diet.

Now we've all passed the gluten free section in the supermarket and seen how small it is. Not only that, the food looks about as appetizing as the packing boxes the food arrives in. This can be distressing in itself, you wander around in a daze, and become very upset and despondent coming to the conclusion you can't eat anything. You leave the supermarket feeling panicky and want to give up and not face the problem.

In a second scenario. You feel happy there are gluten free products and you go crazy buying the bread, biscuits and pizza bases. You thank your lucky stars the nice Mr. Supermarket man has stocked up on this food you can eat, and you rush home with hope life is finally swinging to your advantage.

Now, both scenarios are not as clear cut as you think. In fact the first scenario is better than the second. Why? If the food is available, then no problem. Right? Not exactly. And I'll explain why.

Although the first scenario is distressing, in the long run you will be better off because you will be forced to cook everything from scratch. By doing this, you will eat healthy, and there will be no nasties in there that can make your anxiety worse. In fact, cooking from scratch will improve your health, and likewise, reduce the amount of anxiety you are experiencing. Where the second scenario looks great on the surface, and easier, all those lovely foods you purchased might actually make you feel worse. Primarily because of the amount of sugar and additives that are in them. As I have explained, sugar is distressing on an already stressed out system, so by adding more stress, you will get more symptoms which will make you think something is wrong, and you end up in a loop of more debilitating thoughts. This is another downward spiral, and it's very hard to get your head together when your body is giving you signals things are not right. – But of course things are right, it's just you are feeding your system the kind of food it isn't able to deal with, and hence the feelings.

You may experience the following:

○ Dizziness.

○ Confusion.

○ Chest pains.

○ Tightness in chest.

○ Bloating.

○ Wind.

○ Indigestion.

○ Sickness.

○ A feeling of not feeling well.

○ Anxiety.

○ Shaking.

○ Panic attacks.

○ Depression.

The feelings can be pretty extreme, which tells your mind to hit the alarm bells, and you end up cycling from feeling pretty awful to full blown panic attacks. And all because of the food you are consuming. Take away the stress on your body, and you not only reduce the anxiety, but you can heal physically and mentally, so improving your life in all areas.

Dairy intolerance

This quite often comes part and parcel with gluten intolerance, but luckily we have alternatives that cause no problems, like, rice, soya, and almond milk. Rice is my personal favourite because its light, tastes good, and you can cook with it really easily. Cheese, you can look to goat's cheese in hard block or soft format, and again, tastes good and cooks well.

Butter? - Soya butter is a great alternative and contains 75% less fat, so is better for you.

Ice cream lover? – Don't despair there is a yummy alternative made from soya which most supermarkets stock.

So, so far so good, things are looking up, and the alternatives are making life not so bad, it's all about adapting but you'll quickly get used to it. And at the end of the day, you'll be much healthier for changing your diet.

So where do you start from here?

Bread

Bread is something that plays a big part in our daily diet, and I urge you to make your own. It tastes fabulous, doesn't have any nasties in it, and you can have fresh bread when you want it. Does this sound like a lot of hard work? Maybe you can't face it because you feel so dreadful. I understand, I have been there, and it takes a lot of courage, but I can promise you this, it will get easier over time. And like everything I have shown you in this book, time and patience is one of the areas you will have to persist with. Because the more frustrated you become with the process, the more you fuel the panic. This is about stepping back and allowing the symptoms to wash over you. Don't fight the anxiety. Just allow.

But I digress. So the first thing to do is purchase yourself a bread maker with a gluten free setting. The internet is great for this, so check the reviews and buy yourself the best you can afford. Alternatively check for a second hand one if money is tight. But know in your heart this is one of the best purchases you will make. My current bread maker takes about three hours to make a gluten free loaf, after, I leave the bread to cool, slice, and pop it in a bag and then straight into the freezer. Take what you need, when you need it, works best because the flours in these breads will dry out very quickly and then the bread is more likely to fall apart. I toast mine then place some chicken and maybe a bit of salad to make a toasted sandwich. Or perhaps some goats cheese and some chilli sauce.

And it doesn't have to stop there either. You can make biscuits, waffles, pastry. Anything with a little bit of thought and practice. Check out some books on gluten free dairy free cooking, and you'll soon discover, being intolerant to some foods is not that much of a problem as perhaps you first thought.

Tricks of the trade:
○ Use Bach flower Rescue Remedy to relieve stress and calm your mind.

○ Imagine yourself coping in the situation beforehand.

○ Always congratulate yourself for coping; convince yourself you can handle this.

○ Remember, nobody will think the worse of you if you need to dash to the toilet.

○ Don't be afraid to tell people you suffer.

○ A lot of it is you don't want people finding out.

○ Watch what you eat, knowing your stomach won't cramp will build confidence.

○ Confidence goes a long way to beating I.B.S.

Avoid:

○ Very spicy food.

○ Fried and greasy food.

○ Excess alcohol.

○ Milk and cheese if you are intolerant. Try rice milk and reduce cheese intake if you still crave it. (*Try hard or soft goats cheese, it's a great tasty alternative*).

○ Foods and drink which encourage abdominal gas, e.g. fizzy drink.

○ Instead of shop bought, why not make your own gluten free bread?

Anything else?

Another good idea is to eat little and often, this is especially true when working out the foods that are disagreeable. You don't want to eat an eight course meal then be wondering which were bad, it isn't going to work. And chances are, too much will have the same outcome as something you can't handle. So remember, eat small, make notes, feel the benefits.

Alcohol??

Sorry, but this is a stimulant, not to mention contains a high sugar content. What I said about caffeine runs true for alcohol, use sparingly if you must, but be careful. A few mere sips when sensitive can send you off into the pits of an attack, be strong and steer clear, but that can bring on another problem. Other people.

Don't ask me why, but when you're a non drinker, it seems to offend some people who are. Saying things like, 'go on, take one. What's wrong with you?'

You feel embarrassed. Maybe you don't want to admit you suffer from panic attacks, which might open up a whole host of explaining. But take responsibility for yourself. Stand up and say for health issues you can't. Don't crumble in a moment of weakness, because the only person you'll be harming is yourself. And anyhow, soon enough they'll be too drunk to remember. And if you took the beer, you could be ill for days. - Walk away, and remember you're the important one here, drink is only drink, it doesn't make you a better person for downing umpteen pints. It certainly makes you lighter on money, and far worse health wise.

There's a lot of hype and social acceptance built round this age old drink, yet don't feel you have to be part of it if you're going to suffer. Just take a look around and notice how many kids drink alcohol. Glamorisation from mediums such as films, added with the fact you can't drink by law until a certain age, seems to make them drink younger. But that's not the most damaging part. We are currently in an age of binge drinking, where instead of a steady intake, the drinker consumes as much as possible on a Saturday night shocking the body and harming the liver. Like all things, balance is required, luckily alcohol we can live without.

Sugar

Raw sugar seems to make it into a lot of our food if we like it or not. Basically, the natural sugar you find in fruit is okay in moderation, the body can break this down, the bigger problem comes with the refined sugar that has nothing of worth in it. And it's this stuff the body finds hard to break down causing stress on the system. It's best avoided, or at least greatly reduced, not only because it will help reduce anxiety and panic attacks, but because it diminishes the chance of developing diabetes.

How does it affect us?

Normally, sugar alone doesn't set off panic, but it can cause sweating, light headiness, nervousness, confusion, and a shot of energy which could make you worry into an attack. But make no mistake, we do need a certain amount of sugar, glucose is our brains fuel after all. So like other stimulants, moderation is the order of the day. Yet try not to have any before bedtime (e.g. jam and toast) because it won't help your sleep. This can be contributed to waking up in the small hours and going into an attack. The sugar has found its way through the gut and hey presto! A shot of high speed rocket fuel.

This only lasts for a short period, after which, the body has to work hard to break the sugar down, causing tiredness, lethargy, and a feeling of being less able to cope.

But I can't live without sugar!

If that's the case, have you tried fructose? This is a natural sugar made from fruits, making it a good alternative. The body will have little difficulty in breaking this down, and so won't cause the after-effects refined sugar brings.

Quick Guide

Fresh vegetables and fruits, (especially citrus fruits) are an excellent source of Vitamin C. We need this replenishing daily as our adrenal glands, which produce adrenaline during an attack, uses up our resources.

Protein and complex carbohydrates. Because you use up more protein and complex carbohydrates when under stress, it's good to eat poultry, fish, and whole grain products such as brown breads and cereals. Avoid refined flours as these aggravate your stress response.

Water. Try to drink plenty of water during the day. This flushes the system, and rids of any toxins that have built up over time. Sparkling water introduces gas to an already volatile stomach, so is best avoided for now.

Herbal teas. If you are suffering from heartburn, stomach discomfort, or wind, a useful trick is to sip peppermint or chamomile tea. These have proved countless times a great calmer. Otherwise you might like to try peppermint capsules available from your local health food shop.

Juicing. I mention it here because this is something I came to later in my healing journey and now I can feel the benefits. Vegetable juices, made fresh by using a juicing machine, has enabled me to feel healthier, have more energy, and put my mind at rest that I am doing something highly beneficial for my body. Check it out online and you will be amazed at the kind of things avid juicers have healed themselves from.

Mentally. Watch what you are thinking. Excess worry will cause your stomach to go into fight or flight mode, (excess acid), and with it the uncomfortable symptoms. This is an area you will have to work on, but just keep reassuring yourself everything will be okay, and use meditation which will be of benefit here. Gradually you will calm the stomach just by thinking calmer, but if you still have excess gas and heartburn, check your diet, because something is upsetting your system.

And to sum up?

I guess the bottom line is eat healthily. Steer clear of excess fat, salt and sugar. Refuel correctly, and the attacks won't drain you of your vital nutrients which otherwise lead to fatigue and even more stress. And another thing, remember to eat little and often, and carry something with you like a banana and some dried fruit at all times. Not eating will bring low blood sugar and the dizziness that can trigger an anxiety attack because you worry something is wrong with you. Eat well, and it goes a long way to beating this disorder.

Summary

Tick

Box

☐Eat at sensible times and regularly.

☐Try not to eat just before bedtime. But if you do, eat something light.

☐Breakfast is the most important meal of the day. No myth. Otherwise you're running on empty gas tanks.

☐Cut down on sugar/salt intake. Reduce your alcohol

---

consumption, or stop drinking altogether.

☐Drink plenty of water.

☐Discover any foods which don't agree with you.

☐Consider taking a good quality multi-vitamin.

☐Eat a balanced diet and omit any junk food.

☐Eat vitamin C enriched foods.

☐Try peppermint tea or capsules to calm the stomach.

☐Tepid water with a slice of lemon in the morning cleans out the digestive system. Also calms upset stomachs

☐Try a gluten free dairy free diet. Talk it over with your doctor if you are worried.

☐Buy yourself a breadmaker with a gluten free setting.

☐The internet and books are a great source for gluten free recipes.

☐Don't allow yourself to run on empty because it will bring anxiety symptoms. (Blood sugar drop).

☐Carry food with you at all times. Dried fruit is ideal.

☐Consider juicing fresh fruit/vegetables to bring your body to optimum health and reduce the anxiety. Check out Jason Vale and Joe Cross on the internet for more info.

☐Watch Joe's DVD *'Fat Sick and Nearly Dead.'* An awe-inspiring film about juicing and regaining control over your health.

☐'YOU ARE SAFE.'

- 13 -

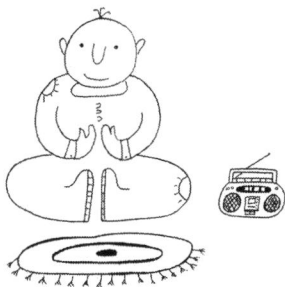

Visualisation & Meditation

Power of the mind

Our very first experience of visualisation comes by way of dreams when we sleep. Small awkward stories, or impossible acts that seem to fizzle from our minds when we wake. But some are so real, so good in fact, we want it to go on. Or sometimes we are unaware we are dreaming at all because it seems that real.

The truth is, the mind can't differentiate between reality and dreams. Put yourself back in a happy time of your life, and you'll feel happy, and sad...

So visualisation can be helpful in calming our minds. Think miles of golden sandy beaches, tall palm trees that waft overhead in the cooling breeze, and blue cloudless skies, and you can't help but relax.

Though you might say, I have no imagination, I can't possibly visualise. But everyone can in one form or another. It might come in short stills to begin with, but the very act of just trying makes a difference. And like all things, practice makes perfect.

But if you are still stuck, luckily we have some help to make things easier.

Narrated meditation tapes/CD's/MP3's

The type I found most beneficial, not only incorporated soothing sounds in the background, but a narrator who picture's the scene. In fact, someone just saying relax over and over again in a certain tone, can have amazing results. It's rather like being in the presence of somebody who is naturally calm, yet, there they are, on tape, and whenever you want them. Which just leaves you to close your eyes, listen, and let everything gently go.

Fighting the panic will only make you more conscious of what's going on inside. The pains, the thoughts, is this going to work?

Granted, the first few times might be an experience you'd rather not have. It's difficult to relax, and there might be some uncomfortable tension here. But ever so slowly, but surely, the grasp anxiety holds over you shall weaken.

Only a small bit of advice here. Find a good selection. Some you might have trouble with. Like the gushing sounds of waterfalls make you opt for the nearest toilet, or, the voice might get on your nerves so much you'd rather not bother. So instead of reducing angst, it actually increases it, killing the whole purpose of visualisation.

And as we are all different. Our tastes, moods, change over time, a CD that might have been good once, holds little power later on. Which means I can't say, get such and such a CD, because of this very fact I've just described. Only you can decide this. Choose the one that suits you at the moment.

And once you have your CD, and are happy with it, use it as desired. You might want to use it before breakfast, again at lunch, and finally before bed. It's entirely your choice. But let me just say. However comfortable you may feel, keep on using this method, because it's a great way of relieving the days stress. After all, stress reduction is the name of the game here. We reach our dreams because we know it will make us happy, and you never get a truly happy person with major anxiety problems.

Where do I find such CD's?

If you find it difficult to get to the shops, don't despair, again these CD's are readily available over the internet. There are sites where you can download the recording into your computer for immediate use. Just because you can't get out, it doesn't mean you won't get to the aids you require in our modern age. Many of mine where ordered over the net and I received them within 1-2 working days. So please, don't feel it's impossible. The products are a mouse click away. Amazon readily stock a large collection, and so do the majority of alternative healing outlets. Not to mention sites such as itunes for digital download.

Tense??

In the extreme, anxiety brings tensions within the body. At best, they are intolerable, at worse, they scare you. Then there are thoughts linked to them like in the following:

Symptom

Tightening of the chest

Thought

'I'm going to have a heart attack. I'm going to die.'

Symptom

Pressure in the head.

Thought

'I've got a brain tumour. I'm going mad.'

It's surprising, but these kind of damaging thoughts might pass through your mind a hundred times a day. The result? They empower to the point where a mere single thought brings with it symptoms, when otherwise you could have been feeling okay.

So instead of saying those to yourself, replace them with:

'These symptoms are created by anxiety alone. There is nothing to fear as I relax in the knowledge I am safe.'

If need be, repeat this a hundred times a day, and take a few minutes for the following visualisation exercise. I've kept it simple but effective, because I know how difficult it can be to concentrate when in an anxiety riddled state.

'I want you to stand in the middle of your room. Take your shoes and socks off and stand tall. Now close your eyes and imagine a beam of golden light entering the crown of your head. Feel the universe energy powering up your being. Relax, you are receiving the ultimate charge.'

Stay like this for five minutes or more. Feel the massive surge of energy through every cell in your body, and don't forget to breathe steadily.

Note: If for any reason you can't stand, it's perfectly okay to do this in the seated position.

Good. Now relax. Take a few deep breaths and clear your mind

'Imagine all the fluids in your body are sinking downwards. Feel the liquid running within you towards the ground. Feel the sensation trickling, and as you do, release all the

tensions you have been holding. Let the muscles go one by one starting from your head. Keep this up for a further five minutes.'

So now you've tried a couple of exercises, how do you feel? Hopefully you'll be quietly surprised exactly how powerful visualisation can be. I'm not claiming you'll be better immediately, because like everything, this will need working on. But put the time in, and you'll begin to notice a difference in your overall anxiety levels.

I can't focus!

Your concentration will be a major factor where the success of your visualisation is concerned. A few minutes can seem a long time when feeling unwell. So the key is, start small, and slowly extend the time. Try starting with five minutes visualization extending to ten when you feel more comfortable. Eventually this will advance to half an hour and then forty-five minutes.

I recommend a forty minute session because it gives you enough time to relax, and stay in that relaxation for a reasonable period of time. By doing this, it reminds your body what it feels like to be tension free, and slowly the period of feeling calm will extend until it becomes a normal state for you.

Which is why visualisation plays such a large part in your recovery programme. Yes, you may feel uneasy right now, but try and use it to good effect. Especially alongside all the other aspects I have shown you.

Dealing with other people's emotions

Powerful as they are, have you ever wondered why sometimes you walk into a room feeling upbeat, only to leave under a cloud of depression because a person made you feel that way?

The answer being, you've tuned into that person's negative emotions and have taken them onboard as your own. Okay, you might have been lending a helpful ear to that person, but the energy passed through the air and soon enough you were down in the hole with them. – In short, what you need is a barrier, and a sturdy one at that.

I'm not saying you're going have to turn into a heartless being with no concern apart from yourself. After all, we are all here on this planet to grow, and by helping other people, that's one way of doing this. What I'm saying is. Listen, help, but don't take it on board. You can do this a number of ways, but this is one of the simplest.

The hooded cloak

'Imagine you're putting on an overly thick cloak. Sweep the material around your shoulders and remember to button up the heavy clasps right underneath your chin. Now take the hood and place it over your head.'

Say: *'I ask the highest being for protection.'*

Gain protection by doing the above exercise. Do this once in the morning, and once before you go to bed. Or if you are about to enter a situation you know will affect you in this way.

You are working hard to sort through your own personal emotions here, and I'm proud of you for doing this. - So please, as cold hearted as it might sound now, don't go trying to sort other people's problems by absorbing theirs as well. It won't do you any good. In fact, you could feel worse, and be left wondering why this has happened. I've done it too many times and it's not pleasant. Empathise for them by all means, yet walk away without churning their problems over and over. The power of other people's problems can overwhelm you, and as you have too many as it is, there simply isn't the space for any more.

'If you are still thinking about a person and their problems half an hour later, you are stuck in their problems.'

Try: - *'Imagine shrinking the person down and placing them in a jam jar. Now put this jam jar on a shelf and walk away. You can always come back to them; it just means you won't be affected when you leave.'*

What if a family member is deeply negative?

As an added extra, try putting that person inside a pink bubble. Pink, being the colour of unconditional love, can help dissipate feelings of negativity and anger. Every time you see them carry out this exercise, and over time, their negativity shall diminish.

You can also do this if you suddenly find yourself in a conflict or confrontation. Visualise a pink bubble around that person and their anger will wane.

To sum up:

O Meditation teaches your body how to relax. It also calms a stressed mind removing the symptoms of anxiety.

O It takes time and practice to master, but persevere, as the results will be worth it.

O Meditate at least once a day, but twice a day will bring faster results.

O This is a powerful tool. Stick with it even if you are finding it difficult at first.

Summary

Tick

Box

☐There is nothing to fear from visualisation, you do it all the time.

☐Narrated meditations are best; use them to help dispel your anxiety.

☐You can buy CD's or download them on an MP3 player.

☐Use these simple exercises everyday and feel the difference.

☐Protect yourself from other people's emotions by using the hooded cloak technique.

☐Put a negative person in a jam jar so they don't affect you.

☐Place a foe in a pink bubble to zap their negativity.

☐Although visualisation is not a quick fix, it will have lasting benefits in the long term.

☐Make time to visualise and meditate.

☐Stick with it, the benefits will come.

☐'YOU ARE SAFE.'

- 14 -

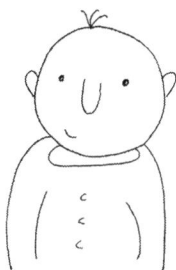

Hypnotherapy

Inspired Therapies

Further along my own healing journey I was lucky enough to meet Eleanor Porter of Inspired Therapies based in Rollesby, Norfolk. Eleanor agreed to help me combat my anxiety with hypnotherapy, and the results have been amazing. So much so I wanted her to explain exactly what she does so you can decide whether this is an avenue you'd like to take. Eleanor kindly agreed to write a piece for the book to describe her methods, and I urge you to investigate this type of healing because the benefits have been extremely positive.

Eleanor was not only kind enough to work through the particular problems I was dealing with, and as result, where surfacing as anxiety, but also record some hypnotherapy tracks so I could go home and work on myself. And I think this an important part to mention here. The therapist will give you all the tools to aid you in your own recovery, but it will be up to you to implement them fully. Yet the hard work pays off, and you will sense a new confidence in your mind and body, as the period of anxiety falls away and you begin to get a hold on your life once again.

So I just want to thank Eleanor for being there and helping me through some of my darkest hours. She is very gifted and I feel very blessed she was there shining a light for me to follow.

Hypnotherapy for anxiety and depression

When Richard asked me to write a piece on hypnotherapy treatment for people suffering from panic attacks and depression, I thought it was a great idea. The responsibility of doing it justice without sounding clinical or terrifying has however, proved far greater than I imagined. Client's that have come to me in the past with anxiety and depression, whether it be for hypnotherapy, or herbal medicine, arrive with the same question. Will this be the one that works, will I achieve 'normality,' or am I destined to travel this road alone? No one can walk in your shoes and feel the emotions that you feel on a daily basis, but a really good therapist should offer to walk with you for part of the way, until you are strong enough to travel the rest of the journey on your own.

The best advice I can give you is to find a therapist that you can truly relate to. I ask my client's to be completely honest with me even about the darkest of thoughts that they are too scared to share with their families or friends. So if you find it difficult to open up to one therapist, don't give up, keep on looking. And once you have found a hypnotherapist that you are completely comfortable with, then you are ready to start your journey into the wonders of your subconscious mind.

Although I would like to say at this stage that hypnotherapy for anxiety and depression is not a quick fix solution. There is no magic formula that fits all, and for me, as a therapist, to understand your thought processes and emotions that govern your day to day life, can be a process of investigation. A process of working through years of experiences, and in some cases, deep trauma's that have been buried but not forgotten.

I appreciate this all sounds quite scary, but remember, your hypnotherapist will guide you through these memories helping you to observe them rather than reliving the pain until resolved.

The first obstacle I tend to experience is the ability for clients to relax. Being unable to switch off the stress and tension from the day, and relax enough to get a good night's sleep, is actually quite common for anyone with responsibilities. But for some, it's the foundation of the nightmare known as anxiety and depression. So be open to 'having a go,' and you may even surprise yourself how easily it comes with practice.

The next point to note is that when you are hypnotised you are not sent to sleep, or in a trance like state where your therapist feeds your subconscious mind with suggestions that would be alien to it. We do talk of 'putting you under,' but this is merely a deeper state of relaxation.

To explain this further, imagine you're a passenger in the car and it's a long journey. You are sitting in the back and not included in the conversation going on in the front, although you can hear it going on. Your mind starts to drift, and your eyes close, giving the appearance you are asleep. You can still hear the conversation and the traffic noises, you are still aware of being in the car, and if someone talks to you, you are able to reply. Well, that is a state of relaxation, and the first stage of hypnosis. Time travels, noises and words can be heard, and the conscious mind is still thinking, but you are relaxed.

Your therapist will then deepen that relaxation and you will still be able to hear everything she says to you. In fact, your subconscious mind is attuned to her voice, and is storing all the positive suggestions made.

It is usually at this point, that I need to differentiate between the hypnotherapy that I offer, and stage hypnosis used for pure entertainment. I can assure you only 4-5% of the human population can be hypnotised to such an extent that they would willingly humiliate themselves on stage. This approach is never adopted by a hypnotherapist as they are offering you therapy not entertainment. So rest assured that will not happen to you.

For peace of mind I always discuss my approach with my clients prior to hypnosis, so that there are no surprises during the treatment, and its due to this consultation technique, I never use a script. The reason being, I like my treatment sessions to be governed by the client, and the only way I can assess the success of my suggestions, is to be constantly watching my client for little signs of stress or deeper relaxation.

During a hypnotherapy consultation we will talk about you for about an hour, and it is this information that governs your hypnosis. Each hypnotherapist will approach the hypnosis differently, but I start by suggesting my clients create a safe room in their minds. A place where you can go when you are scared or stressed, it offers a safe place where no one else can go. From here we can focus on the present day, how you feel, and accentuate the positive aspects of your life. The reason you get up in the morning whether that is your work, family, friends, or a desire to beat this disorder, it does not matter. Hypnotherapy should be about boosting confidence, resilience, and self esteem in all aspects of your life that have been destroyed or diminished by someone, or something, in the past.

Rebuilding each of these emotional aspects of a client is a slow process, but as progress is made, I then start to introduce negative aspects from before. This may be an event, a lifestyle, or a person who has contributed to the clients current emotional state, and we take those negatives and build positive images from them. We view trauma's as if you were watching from the outside looking in, and in case of childhood issues, I use regression to return to the exact trauma and allow you the client to resolve the issues. This is always done in a positive way and so boosting confidence and self esteem.

As I said before, there is no solution that fits all, and every treatment should be based on how the client feels at that particular moment in time, and not the next stage of the healing process because we all have good and bad days.

The wonderful aspect of hypnotherapy, is quite often the trauma or event that we believe is governing our future, can sometimes be overshadowed by other events. The very same ones we have forgotten because they are so trivial to us at the time. So be prepared to be surprised at you own resilience, a fact that sometimes can be lost when struggling with the symptoms of anxiety.

In summary, with the right hypnotherapist and positive attitude towards your own healing path, hypnotherapy can be insightful, positive, constructive, and cathartic, as well as surprising and rewarding. Those who say it does not work are those that are too scared to try it for themselves. So why not trust in your own intelligence and try to understand and embrace your past to make a positive difference to your future.

I wish you every success, and I hope my introduction to hypnotherapy has encouraged you to take the first step towards your recovery. - Good luck.

Eleanor Porter 2014 - Visit: www.inspired-therapies.co.uk

-15-

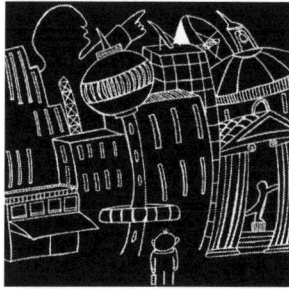

To walk the Devil's Yard

'Remedy to take is <u>Elm</u>. Helps keep things in perspective. Keeps inner confidence and gives ability to cope. Add to Rescue Remedy.'

As you know by now my first major panic attack happened at the cinema, and because of this, I found the situation totally unbearable. If somebody asked, 'would you like to go and see the latest blockbuster?' I'd immediately feel the panic build and there was nothing I could do but decline. The whole scenario had smashed my confidence into tiny pieces, and to walk the Devil's yard would have been impossible.

The Devil, (namely Panic), would surely have noticed my return for some more nerve bashing, and he wouldn't have thought twice about delivering. But that wasn't a single case with the cinema. Whenever an attack happened, it stopped me from going where the episode had taken place. Slowly but surely, I was fast becoming a lone prisoner held within boundaries set by my own mind. To roll over and then give up, well, it's not hard to see where I would have ended. A single room. Too scared to come out, I would have suffered badly, unable to operate and just waiting to die.

CONSEQUENCE OF AVOIDENCE

PANIC ATTACK

⇊

THOUGHT: 'I MUST AVOID SITUATION'

⇊

SUCCESSFUL AVOIDANCE

⇊

ACTIVITIES RESTRICTED

⇊

PANIC ATTACK

⇊

THOUGHT: 'I MUST AVOID SITUATION'

⇊

SUCCESSFUL AVOIDANCE

⇊

ACTIVITIES RESTRICTED

⇊

AND SO ON

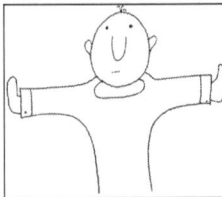

A sad state of affairs, and this is not an uncommon scenario. Panic puts real fear into us. Our thinking says, 'if we go and do so and so, will an attack strike?' But even worse, before you fully realise the feelings are there, you sense you're sitting on the edge of a rock face with your feet dangling over the edge. God, one move, and it's good night Vienna.

So how can we overcome these false alarms? What can you do now to change the process, so again you can walk wherever you want, go and see whatever you desire, and heck, do whatever you damn well want? – Well, read on, this is important.

Rewriting your personal hard drive

Rather like a new computer we buy from the store, from the outset we too come with very little programming. We have to learn through our elders the correct way of dealing with people, and generally how the world works. Then, later we learn a trade, and information is stored at a slightly slower pace than our childhood years. Which is the reason why, whatever happened to us early on, has a dramatic influence on how we deal with life today. But saying that, a trauma that's happened recently, can also create problems, and will need to be dealt with so you can leave it behind and move forward.

To do this, just like you clear the rubbish out of your computer, you need to clear the rubbish out of your mind so you can rewrite your own hard drive.

Although we can't download a new programme from an internet site, save it to disc, then load the new information into our brains, we can change it by utilising several powerful techniques. These include, affirmations, visualisation, desensitisation, and flower remedies. Used together, they will break the panic, and bring confidence so anxiety will never strike again.

Reprogramming your mind

JUNK   CLEAN   NEW INSTALL

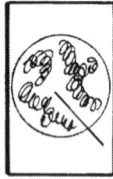

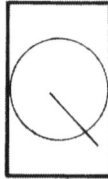

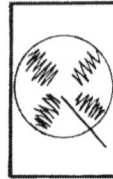

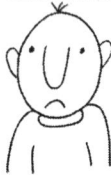

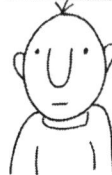

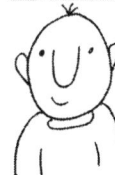

How can I change this?

Because you've labelled a situation as a no go area, and to be avoided at all costs, your hard drive has been written and there's an association with panic here. Just thinking of the situation starts the fear. And that's without actually going near the place. So, by re-writing, or in other words, proving to yourself you can deal with it, the hard drive will be cleaned, and a new programme of positive will dissociate the panic from the problem area. This allows you your freedom back. In principle, it's that's easy.

So where do we go from here?

What I'm going to do now, is take you through the four stages, so you'll be able to control any given situation you are currently having problems with. But firstly, you will need to do the preparation step; this is highly important and will make a world of difference in the success of the exercise.

To walk the Devil's Yard
4 step action plan

1.Pre-Run Situation in Your Mind

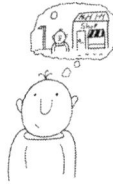

2.Visit Situation (use FRT table)

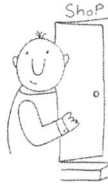

3.Evaluate Situation (use PAT table)

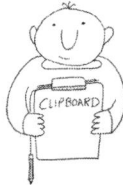

4.Revisit Situation Stronger than before

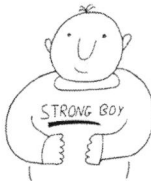

But please, don't become despondent if things don't move as fast as you'd like. Be patient with yourself and this exercise. It's extremely powerful and persistence does pay off.

The Three Step Preparation Plan

○ Take Rescue Remedy at least the day prior to undertaking this exercise.

○ Practice controlled breathing.

○ Take a few minutes out and calm the mind with positive affirmations.

De-sensitise – Breaking the anxiety barrier

Stage 1 – The Pre-Run Visualisation

I want you to think of a situation you panic in. Something that can be tried and evaluated many times, without being too far from where you live. For examples sake, I'm going to pick visiting the local newsagent for some milk and a loaf of bread.

Now do the following;

○ Take Rescue Remedy.

○ Practice controlled breathing.

○ Take a few minutes and calm the mind with positive affirmations.

○ Say: *'I can do this; I am getting stronger by the minute.'*

○ Keep the reassuring going, before, and during the actual event itself.

○ You can do this.

○ You are safe.

Good. Now visualise in your mind's eye, every step from leaving the room you're in, all the way to returning from the shop with the goods in your hands. For help, I'm going to show you how.

Say: *'I am getting stronger by the minute.'*

Going shopping – Visualisation exercise

You leave the kitchen and walk down the hall, you pick your house keys up from the small table with the telephone on, and you proceed to the coat hooks. You lift your coat off and put it on; making sure your money is in the pocket, and your Rescue Remedy is there in case you need it.

Satisfied everything is in order, you confidently open the front door and step outside. You close the door and lock it, a couple of wiggles on the handle just to make sure.

Say: *'I am feeling strong today, I can do this.'*

You turn and begin to walk in the direction of the shops. You see your neighbour coming and you smile. You comment on what a nice day it is. Your neighbour repays the pleasantries and you keep going, making sure not to rush because there is all the time in the world.

The shop is coming up on your right, but you have to cross the road to get to it. You stop at the pavements edge and look both ways before crossing the road.

Say: *'The shop holds no fear for me, I am strong.'*

Safely the other side, you calmly enter the shop, which already has a couple of people in it. A young man is over the back reading a magazine, whilst an elderly lady is having difficulty in finding the correct change for the man behind the counter.

You walk over to the bread stand in the far corner and pick up a fresh loaf. Beside the stand is the refrigerator, which you open and take out a pint of milk. You close the door and head for the cashier.

Say: *'I have all the time in the world, I am safe.'*

The old lady has just dropped all her coins on the floor and is trying her best to retrieve them. You tell her not to worry, and kindly bend over and scoop up the change. You hand her the money, and she smiles and thanks you. Subsequently you can't help but feel warm inside.

The old lady leaves, and you pay for your goods and exit the shop.

You cross the road and walk back towards your house. This time a young woman stops you to ask the time, which you kindly oblige. She says thanks, and you follow the same path and arrive at your front door.

Feel proud of yourself and say: *'I am stronger today.'*

You put the goods down, unlock the door, pick the goods up, and walk in closing the door behind. You go through to the kitchen and put the goods on the work surface. You congratulate yourself on a task well done.

And there you have it. By visualising, it not only takes much of the fear away, but if you do find yourself becoming more anxious, you can control it that much better in an environment where you feel safe.

Tip: *'Try recording this example or your own version on tape. By giving yourself something to listen to, this will allow you to visualise the task that bit easier.'*

Remember to do the following after:

O Take Rescue Remedy.

O Control your breathing.

O Use positive affirmations.

O Self congratulate.

O Take some time to sit back and relax.

There's no limit to the number of times you can carry this out, but obviously, when you're comfortable with this stage it's time to move onto the practical exercise. But don't be tempted to miss the visualisation out, because it's an important part of the process. As I explained in the previous chapter, the mind is affected by thought and reality, it can't differentiate between the two. So doing this is the same as carrying out the real thing where it's concerned.

'By programming your mind, you are not only telling yourself you are safe, but also strong enough to cope.'

Stage 2 – Visit the Situation

Before I explain this stage, I need to introduce you to one of the tools you'll be using throughout this part of the exercise; it's called the Feelings Record Table, or F.R.T. This allows you to keep a record of your progress, build further affirmations, and remind yourself how far you've come. But remember, however little the progress you make, be pleased with yourself here, you are doing something incredibly brave that many people would shy away from. Instead, they'd rather put up with the panics and feelings of sickness. But you are doing it, and for this reason alone you should be extremely proud of yourself.

The Feelings Record Table (FRT)

Date	Task	Feelings	Why?	Severity
18/2/02	Shopping	Felt anxious, a bit sick, and light headed.	I fear if an attack will strike.	6/10

All common symptoms, but notice the 'Why?' column. It consists of one thought, the fear of having a panic attack. But that thought alone can then lead to more drastic thinking, like, what's wrong with me, I feel strange. Thus feeding the feelings. It's a vicious circle syndrome. (See panic loop). Because the more negative thoughts you have, the worse they become, and this builds a mental monster for you. Remain positive, and recognise the feelings for what they are.

The trick here is...

1. Recognise what you are doing to yourself.

2. Re-address this through altered thinking.

3. Try the whole situation again.

The Positive Affirmation Table (PAT)

Now examine this table:

*Positive	#New affirmation
(Turn negative from FRT table to positive)	
*These sensations are of panic, it is a natural response.	
# *'I am fit and healthy. There is nothing wrong with me, & I relax in the knowledge I will overcome this.'*	

By reversing our thoughts from negative to positive, it removes the fear something is wrong. It's rather like someone saying, 'it's okay, there's nothing to worry about.' And you know from personal experience, when a person says that, it has an overall calming effect upon you.

Sadly, positive self talk is not a 'click your fingers and I'm fixed' kind of deal. What it is though, is a highly effective method of repairing a defective belief system. And not only that, it lasts with you forever.

Yes, you will need to work on this constantly for now, and then have to top it up from time to time in the future. Life after all throws many a quandary our way, but it will serve you well by re-programming your way of dealing with things.

'Only __YOU__ can change your pattern of thinking, nobody else can do it for you.'

What you'll need:

O A small pad.

O A pen or pencil.

O Bach flower Rescue Remedy.

O A strong mind set with positive affirmations. (Write your affirmations on a card and keep them with you).

Get these items together, and whenever you feel panicky, take some Rescue Remedy and control your breathing. Also, not forgetting to say the affirmations on your card.

I can't say this enough times, but keep this up, and it will make all the difference between success and failure.

You have to want this. You have to be so determined this won't beat you, you'll fight on, no matter how you feel. – But then I know you're not the kind of person to sit down and just give up. I mean, you wouldn't have got this far into the book if you were more interested in throwing in the towel than completing the tasks. So let's start.

Pick something that's not too threatening. I don't want you getting an attack the moment you think of it. Maybe you want to get to the park, take the dog, or meet somebody. Basically, anything that's not too big, but find a little bit of a challenge.

So, take your small note pad and pencil, copy the first table, (FRT), although leave it blank for you to fill in during the task. Pop the two items into your pocket and set out.

And remember:

○ Control your breathing from the outset. Make sure it's kept at an even speed and not strained. Keep it natural. You want to stay away from the rapid short breaths that heighten your sensations.

○ Take the Rescue Remedy. Use every ten minutes if need be, it will help you cope with the situation.

○ Say your affirmations throughout, and keep telling yourself you can do this. You will not come to any harm.

○ Say: *'I am safe.'*

The moment the feelings and thoughts come, however small, jot them down. Keep doing this, and if you happen to feel you can't go any longer, turn around and head home. This is not some kind of endurance test, if you feel really bad move back into a situation where you feel more comfortable. This method is designed to push you gently forward, and although it takes longer, it will be kinder on you.

Once back home do the following:

○ **Add Rescue Remedy to a cool glass of water, sip, and relax.**

○ **Meditate.**

○ **Take a relaxing bath. Add a few drops of Rock Water to the bath for added calm.**

○ **Use some more Rescue Remedy.**

○ **Congratulate yourself.**

STAGE 3 – The Evaluation

Here is an important stage. It's where you look at the feelings and turn them around into the positive. This gives you reassurance everything is okay, and the feelings are triggered by the situation, and not because of any physical defect.

Consult your FRT table and switch to the positive. Now fill the positives into the positive affirmation table (PAT) and make up some positive affirmations for you to say. Read these over and feel good about what you have achieved.

You may find this hard at first. But don't worry, with a little practice it will soon become second nature, and you'll be filling these tables in without any problems at all.

Now do:

○ **Repeatedly read through the positives until you are familiar with them.**

○Try and put yourself in a mindset, that when you enter the same situation again, panic will not be a problem. An attack will not happen.

○Convince yourself panic attacks are a thing of the past. Say, 'I am moving forward.'

STAGE 4 – Revisit the Situation

This can be later in the day if you feel up to it. Or perhaps the next day, it's entirely your choice. But don't leave it too long otherwise all your hard work will go to waste. What we are doing here is pushing your panic envelope. Rather like an athlete who pushes his endurance a step further every time he hits the track, you are pushing your anxiety tolerance. It's the same deal. The more times you do this, the easier it gets.

For me, I sat through Lord of the Rings when I was pushing myself through this. – By the third hour I was getting very uncomfortable. But saying that, the whole experience was worth it. The next film I saw was easier to take, I actually started to think about the story instead of what was going on inside of me, and the films distraction was playing a big part in my recovery too.

So you see, by re-visiting the problem areas, we can actually turn things around. Smile to yourself when the feelings begin to subside a little, because when that happens, you'll know you're well on your way towards recovery.

Congratulate yourself. Write in your diary what a good job you did, and the next time will be even better. And it will. Yes I know it may seem tough. But by pushing yourself a little further each time, it is the best way of proving to your mind you can handle any situation the world hurls in your direction. And eventually, you'll leave your house in the mind set that a panic attack will not happen, because you have everything under control. That kind of thinking will overcome fear. Because fear hits a solid wall of positive, and when it does that, it splinters into tiny pieces where it can do no harm. – Mission successful!

○ Enter exactly the same situation as before.

○ Use the Feelings Record Table. (FRT).

○ Put all negative feelings back into positive. (PAT table).

○ Use your new positive affirmations.

○ Counteract any anxious feelings with Rescue Remedy and controlled breathing etc.

○ Keep repeating exercises until the situation creates little or no fear.

○ Congratulate yourself and then move on to another problem area.

You might feel a certain amount of anxiety in a situation, and it doesn't matter how many times you keep revisiting it, the anxious feelings have got to a certain point but won't fall any lower. Don't get disheartened, because it just means your overall anxiety level needs to be reduced further until a situation becomes fully comfortable. To do this, you'll find by walking the Devil's yard in many situations, the level of discomfort felt will lower, and that will enhance your overall confidence as well. Not to mention, boosting the amount of conviction in your own mind that a situation will not be a problem anymore.

'Every time you start again, you start from a stronger

position than before. Be proud of your achievements, you have made a big step forward.'

I realise it seems hard, and you'll feel like this is all too much at times, but use the flower remedies along with the positive self talk. Think, *'I don't have panic attacks,'* not, *'I fear when the next panic attack will strike.'* Because a lot of the cause is the expectation an attack will happen. And I know they seem out of the blue, one moment you were perfectly fine, and next. Bam! But changing your mind set has a lot of power here. And every tool you can use to ward off, or reduce the symptoms of an attack, is obviously advantageous. But hold in there. Because every time you do this, your world will become that bit easier.

So take your time, be easy on yourself, and know this is all for the better.

Tip: - *'If you are afraid of doing this exercise on your own, take a friend. There's no shame in having some support here.'*

Some things to remember when walking the Devil's Yard

1. First, remember to take your **Rescue Remedy**. If you have seen a **Bach flower practitioner and have a bottle made to suit you**, take that as well. If the anxiety rises, use more often than stated. Every half hour, or at worst, in five or ten minutes intervals.

2. Use your deep breathing technique. **Concentrate on the breath.**

3. Keep telling yourself:

'I have control, this is only panic.'

'It is my mind playing tricks on me.'

'I will not come to any harm.'

'I am Safe.'

4. **Talk to somebody** if the situation allows. Call someone and have a chat. This is an excellent way of turning your **mind away from the panic.**

5. Take a pen and paper with you. **Write the symptoms down** and record on a scale of **0-10** how bad the sensations are. Also, simply by the act of writing, the symptoms subside. **Counteract your feelings with positive ones,** and you'll be amazed with the reality. This is just another panic moment, it will pass.

'As I found through my own experience, it does get easier, persistence does pay off, and it will be worth it.'

Summary

Tick

Box

☐We become over sensitive to situations, especially if a panic attack occurred here.

☐By slowly re-introducing heightening levels of stress, it breaks the panic – The mind recognises it can cope in these situations.

☐Recognise your feelings. Counteract with positive self talk and record tables.

☐Take a friend with you. Or meet them at the destination or after the task.

☐Use Bach flower remedies and relaxation techniques throughout.

☐However small, congratulate yourself on each success.

☐Be patient. This method takes time but is highly effective.

☐Remember, 'YOU ARE SAFE.'

The Wow Factor

So what is the wow factor exactly? The wow factor is self congratulation. Without this we tend to dwell on the things we didn't achieve today, the things that make our lives difficult, and hence why we sink deeper into that hole I've spoken about already.

So instead of saying, 'I'm useless, I couldn't make it around the shop without having a panic attack', say, 'Wow! I got much further this time, I must be getting better.'

Self congratulation is a very crucial part of your journey and your success.

Now let's get it all on paper so you can see how far you've come, and have a point of reference to refer to when you need uplifting. - You must record the triumphs to remind yourself of them. Log everything, however small a success, write it down. That includes everything you have achieved in this book so far, because what you are actually doing here is playing emotional space invaders. Instead of death rays, you're using positive rays, shooting down all those negative invaders.

So from today, congratulate and recognise how far you've come. Don't dwell on the negatives, there are always positives in every situation.

Achievement + Positive Affirmation = Confidence

- 16 -

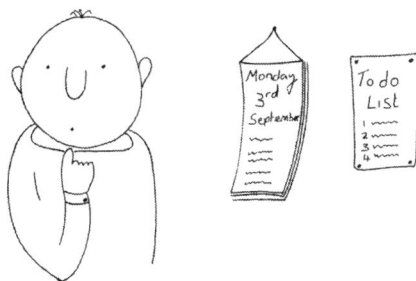

What a difference a Day Makes

We've already tackled individual tasks in the previous chapter, now it's time to look at a whole day. For this, I want you to plan your day more like a military exercise. Set realistic goals and time spans so not to cause exhaustion, stress, and definitely no rush. This might start off with a couple of jobs. Maybe you need to visit the supermarket for instance, and say, the library. Tackle one in the morning, and the other in the afternoon. This way you won't be worrying if you have enough time to complete the tasks you set for that particular day. But just like before, record in a chart format the task, how you felt, and the positives you got out of the whole experience. Remembering self congratulation and Bach flower remedies, not forgetting repeated affirmations such as, *'I am safe'* and any others you may choose.

By introducing a structure to the whole day, you are less likely to panic. You know in your head you have this number of tasks, and nothing else.

So don't go cramming any more in, otherwise you'll be undoing all the good work. Sickness will strike, and the negative thoughts can all too easily creep back in when you're at your weakest.

To quickly summarise this:

○ Break down your day into realistic goals.

○ Don't try and run before you can walk. There is no shame doing one or two tasks in the beginning.

○ As in the chapter, 'To Walk the Devil's Yard,' record all your feelings and counteract with positives.

○ Gradually increase the tasks to a point you feel comfortable. The idea is to do less than you were doing before in a 24 hour period.

○ Controlled structure brings with it less panic.

○ Relax. Use Bach flower remedies, meditate, and remember to control the breath.

○ Congratulate yourself on every achievement, however small that may be.

○ You are safe.

As time and practice progress, the day will become more manageable and so will the number of things you can do. Although always keep a limit. Make time to eat, relax, and talk. I've always found a good DVD does the trick when times are difficult. Music can also transport you to lighter moods and should be utilised whenever possible.

But let's now look deeper into you, let's find out what's really going on that worries you so much panic has set in. And if that sounds a little frightening, it needn't be. I'll take you through steadily, and by the end, you should understand yourself that little bit better.

Current problems

How do you feel about your life? – No really, what areas do you feel are causing you the most aggro that you could well do without?

To make things easier, take a fresh piece of paper and write down your answers under the following headings.

Career

e.g. Is it a job you hate? Too many hours? Somebody at work you don't get along with. Maybe you fell into this work and are unsure how to get out. Perhaps you are lacking employment right now and have low self esteem.

Husband/Wife/Partner

e.g. Deficient in the support side. Feel you are doing all the work in the relationship with no return. Something they do really aggravates you. Maybe they are over protective or highly jealous. Perhaps you feel the love has gone now.

Family

e.g. Mother, father, or both, have little time for you. They criticise whatever you do. You feel as though you are a disappointment. You feel you are not the child they wanted. You find everything you do never pleases them.

Or maybe it's towards your own family, where you feel you haven't spent enough time with them as late. Or you punish yourself because you can't buy what you think they should have. Perhaps you only see them for short periods because of a job or divorce.

Friends

Feelings of drifting away from them. You feel there is no common ground between you anymore and conversation has become false and stilted. Or maybe you are put upon by your friends, such as, 'Good old Bob, he'll put that right for you', or, 'Sue will be able to do that for free, won't you Sue.' And in this situation, you find yourself saying yes, when you really mean **NO!**

Environment

e.g. You don't like where you live. The neighbours are difficult. You feel cut off. You can't relate to those around you. You feel a deep sense of loneliness when alone or surrounded by a group of people.

Money

e.g. Bad debts worry you. You seem to be working hard with nothing to show for it. You want to buy nice things but a lack of cash drags you down. Credit card bills are mounting.

Taking it further

That's good, see how you can recognise where all the problems are coming from? And now with them on paper, it becomes easier to understand why you feel the way you do.

Now try:

O**Why am I fed up today?**

O**Why does my life style make me feel anxious?**

O**How did I get to this point in my life?**

At first glance, you might be thinking my life is more complicated than these questions. But look again, and you'll be surprised how much ground they actually cover. - I'm not trying to simplify your current issues, only simplify the way you look upon them, making this whole process easier.

So start right now and work through them. See if you can recognise any factors, and break them down by putting them in a chart format like the following.

My current belief system

> **I'm overworked, I have no time to do the things I want anymore.**
>
> **I feel trapped in a relationship but I have no way of getting out.**
>
> **I have no money. I will never find enough to get out of this life and lead the one I want.**
>
> **I want to make a difference, but I'll never get a chance.**

This is a simple way of showing what's currently going around your head, and having the negative effect of dragging you down and making you feel awful. For instance, your body shakes when you are angry, now think what happens when such a strong emotion is directed at you, by you, twenty four seven. Because mostly we beat ourselves up. Yes we are angry at family and so forth, but begin by tracking your thoughts and you'll find you're doing an amazing amount of self berating. For example, *'I must be a total loser because I didn't get that job'*, or, *'I hate myself because I can't cope with what normal people cope with.'*

This is harmful and needs to be changed. You are unique, and that's not a nice way of saying you are ugly, stupid, or a waste of space, because in the right mind-set nobody on this planet is any one of those. In this mode we all have a talent, we are all beautiful, and none of us are certainly a waste of space.

So don't go thinking because you have always felt different from others, you must be some kind of freak, because that couldn't be further from the truth. You feel different, because there is a closeness to the present self. You, in your natural state, are fun loving, compassionate, and have big dreams of making a difference. But also, you don't settle for sitting around, you want to be going places and feel true happiness within.

And although it might be hard to believe right now, you actually have a real connection with people. You'll grow to appreciate this more as you progress on the healing journey and realise you are something a bit special.

The Bottom line. You are not a person that should be berated, or in the extreme destroyed. You are you, be proud of who you are and the contribution you bring to the planet called earth.

Stuck in the problem

It's easy to say, 'don't get stuck in the problem.' But exactly how do you un-stick what seems at the time un-stickable? Especially when you dwell on the problem so long it appears there is nothing else you can think about. And the longer you think, the bigger the problem grows, and the more convinced you become it's irreversible. But it is. The trick here is to step back and look at the whole picture. Not to concentrate on the small glitch that's been troubling you up to now. And in the whole scheme of things, it is a glitch. Something that can be overcome using the following methods:

⭘ Bach flower remedies.

O Positive self talk.

O Talking to a trusted friend.

O Often you can solve a problem by working through it on paper.

O Meditate.

O Hypnotherapy tape.

O Listen to uplifting music to lift the spirit.

O Distract your mind on something nice.

O Think, 'this is not a problem, this is a test for greater inner growth.'

O And remember, the act of actually solving, is far easier than the thought.

But whatever you do, try not to get frustrated. Acknowledge this is something you must deal with, but once over, you'll be able to resume business as usual.

Gain strength within and just do it! Otherwise time will pass, and the regrets you hadn't done anything sooner will creep in.

O Change a problem into an advantage.

O Understand things happen for a reason.

O As hard as a problem seems right now, the reason will become apparent later.

O A problem is a test, but can be overcome.

The stuck feeling comes around because there's an overwhelming sense that hope is all lost. You feel too tired to battle, you want to sit down and give up, you'll probably be angry at the situation, a person, or yourself. And a few others will creep in too. Like not wanting to ask for help and finding it difficult to say no. Which can also lead onto seeking somebody's approval to make you feel better. But fear not, you will become unstuck. And as a tool to help you on your way, try the following remedies:

Elm - Confidence, keeps things in perspective, ability to cope.

Cerato - Inner trust, stick with own convictions.

Gentian - Optimism and trust. Look at potential.

Agrimony - Calm mind, talk things through.

Wild Oat - Feeling of being stuck, unsure what to do with life.

Gives positive direction with clarity.

'Don't stay so long in the past, because the future might have gone before you get there.'

Emotions – Self analysing

So now let's look more into the emotional side. Why do you feel so bad?

Is it:

O Anger?

O Frustration?

O Boredom?

O Tiredness?

Write down how you currently feel inside. Don't miss anything. Really get on paper the emotions you are dealing with, because that will come as a release, along with a better understanding of why you feel the way you do.

For instance, do you feel tearful all the time? Have you noticed this become heightened when thinking or dealing with a particular situation? Or do you feel like screaming out and leaving the situation you are currently in? And why?

For me, I can put a lot down to my self berating. An anger towards myself for not being good enough, unable to cope, and unsure to where my life was exactly going. And so there was a certain amount of frustration because I wasn't where I thought I should be. I was getting older for sure, but I still hadn't progressed any further since leaving school. So as hard as I tried, as tired as I got, I just couldn't bash through and make a success. I was a failure in my own mind, but little did I know inside there was a talent waiting to be harnessed. An ability to write.

But when we have a low self image, we tend to take onboard others' negative opinions of ourselves, and this reinforces our already failing belief system. For examples sake, somebody repeatedly questions you. *'How would anybody fancy that?'* looking you up and down in disgust.

The result? - A stronger case in your own mind you are in fact ugly, and you should be resigned to the scrap heap. This knocks onto a failing confidence, self hatred, and pushing affection away because you feel unworthy.

But what's the point you ask? Why dig into this stuff and make yourself unhappy?

Because, understanding why allows you to re-address the problem. All kinds of negative stuff has happened to you, and because of this, it has scored your personal hard drive giving you a defective belief system.

We are talking heaps of junk other people have imposed upon

you, which you have taken on board as your reality. But no fear, that is all about to change. Today is the beginning for rewriting that hard drive with positive self talk, and bringing back the reality of who you are.

Example: negative

I feel tearful all the time, numb inside because I don't feel like I really belong in this world. People make me feel inadequate, they speak to me rarely, but more often than not they pass me by and speak to somebody better adjusted to the world. I feel so tired of trying and failing. Why can't I be a success, why do people look at me as though I'm nothing, then maybe that's what I am. A Mr. nobody.

Do I feel sadness? All the time. I feel alone, but the thought of company makes my insides turn inside. I feel flushed, I want to escape but to where? Wherever I'd run I'd never be able to run from the problem. Namely me.

A brief example, but it's enough to give you an idea what you have to do. Obviously you'll be writing more and covering different areas as well, but this is a great way of seeing what you are experiencing. Because when you are in the problem and dealing with such varied emotions, it's difficult to verbalise but can be easier to write instead.

○Emotions are funny things, they can make or break you in a moment. By understanding your emotions, you can realise the reasons why you feel the way you do.

○You think negative feelings about yourself through repeated exposure of each problem over a certain amount of time.

○Every negative belief carries with it similar emotions. e.g. anger, frustration, hatred, which can make things more confusing along the way. Through careful deduction, you will be able to pinpoint and eradicate these.

So:

○Rewrite your own belief system through positive affirmations.

○Talk over your problems with a trusted friend.

○Use Bach flower remedies.

○Say: *'Starting from TODAY, I will overcome this.'*

○You are safe.

Another look - So now you have your emotions written down on paper you can address them one by one. But of course, there is the chance some will have been missed. Not a problem, always carry a notepad around with you, and when one springs to mind, simply jot it down. You'll be amazed where, how, and why, you've been affected to such a degree. But don't dwell on each for too long, change to the positive and concentrate on that only. The negative has happened, you can't change that fact, what you can do is change the effect it has upon you.

Change to the positive

Nobody has the right to make me feel inadequate, I am equal to them. They probably don't know what to say to me that's why they pass me by. It's nothing personal.

I am a success, dealing with this I have little success's every day, I am doing well and getting stronger with every moment past.

183

So:

○Realise why you feel the way you do.

○Recognise you can change this.

○Turn it round and stick with it.

○The negative is not who you are, believe in better.

I started this chapter talking about how to control your day, how to survive without panics, and desensitise yourself so the symptoms vanish. Re-evaluating and changing what you feel in life is a key factor also. - And you know what? It's surprising what a difference a day makes.

Summary

Tick

Box

☐Plan your entire day in chart form. Be realistic with what you can achieve.

☐Don't start off with too many tasks. Keep it simple until you get used to this way of anxiety exposure.

☐Use Bach flower Rescue Remedy.

☐Write down how you feel about all the problems you currently have.

☐Understand why you feel the way you do. Recognise the changes that need to be put in place to make your life easier.

☐Stick with the positive and bin the negative.

☐Be easy on yourself.

☐Take time out to relax.

☐Self congratulate.

☐You can cope and get through this.

☐I believe in you.

☐Remember, 'YOU ARE SAFE.'

- 17 -

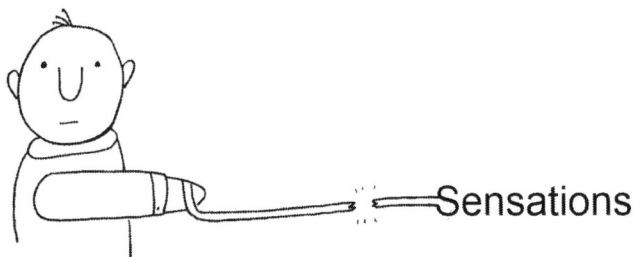

Sensations

Coping Strategies

Dealing with anxiety on a daily basis

This is one of those important areas we need to cover because this is how you cope with your everyday life. When anxiety strikes it can be pretty hard to operate. The thoughts tend to thrash about something bad, and because these heighten your symptoms further, you get locked in a loop of despair, frightening thoughts and physical pain. - So, how do you cope? How do you break the thoughts and feelings to break the cycle???

Now this is an area that takes some training on your part. You have become oversensitive to every twitch, pain, and sensation in your body. In fact, sometimes even without being conscious, your mind is searching for them, even anticipating them, and of course fearing them. And as we know by now, fear fuels the anxiety further, so we must reduce the fear to overcome the anxiety condition. Do this, and we are winning. But like all the exercises I have shown you, it takes time and patience. I'm not talking days, or even weeks, this can take months or even years, but what I can say, is it will get easier over time. You won't feel the debilitating feelings you felt a few weeks ago before you started the programme. Things will progress, and you will have set backs from time to time, but you'll see the fear fall by the wayside as your ability to cope becomes stronger. The more practice you do, the easier you'll find life. And that's the deal.

So while I can't say do this particular thing and you'll cope better right away, I can help you put in place strategies that will teach you how to cope with what you are feeling, and allow you to deal with all of this until eventually everything recedes and normality resumes.

Two areas we need to look at:

◯**The physical feelings.**

◯**The mental aspect.**

Which comes first? To answer this I always think it rather like the chicken or the egg question. Is it the thought that creates the physical feelings? Or is it the Physical feelings that creates the thoughts? Tough one to answer, and I can only go by my own experiences. But I will say this; thoughts are a major driving force.

You think:

◯**I am dying.**

◯**I have a defective heart.**

◯**I am having a heart attack.**

◯**I have something else wrong with me.**

◯**I can't cope.**

◯**If I go outside I will die.**

○I fear the feelings happening again.

○I feel awful.

○I feel I will never be free from anxiety.

○I feel a need to get to hospital.

Now these very same thoughts will happen if you feel the physical symptoms which start the panic loop. Things will quickly get out of hand, and before you know it, you dive headlong into a panic attack. So we need to stick a spanner in the works. We need to stall the panic loop and bring everything back under control. Changing your thought patterns is the key here, but it takes time and effort to perfect this. But perfect this you will.

Coping strategy 101

You are feeling anxious and the physical feelings are becoming distressing. Coping strategies are something we can work on, and the longer you practice, the more effective they will become. Yes you might think I've heard this all before, there is nothing new here, but there is. Repetition and allowing is the answer. Control the panicky thoughts and the long spans of feeling unwell will shorten, your life will return. I promise you this. THERE IS NOTHING YOU CAN'T IMPROVE BY ALTERING YOUR THINKING.'

Self talk

Keep telling yourself you are okay, you are fine and there is nothing wrong with you. Remind yourself your doctor has given you the all clear and you are fit and well.

'These are only symptoms of anxiety and nothing else. You are fine.'

At first you will find this hard, especially during the early days, but keep this up as things will become easier.

'Positive reassurance thinking, along with not feeding fear into a situation, will break the panic.'

Talk with someone

If you are on your own make a phone call. Talk to the person on the other end and rationalize why you are having a panic attack. Talking it over reassures you and will bring the feelings under control.

Rescue Remedy

Add a few drops of remedy to a glass of water and sip regularly.

Other premixed remedies to try: (From creature comforters uk)

Chill Out! – Formulated to help initiate a naturally relaxing process.

Sweet Dreams. - Formulated to help initiate a naturally unwinding process.

Dutch Courage! - Formulated to help initiate a natural confidence.

Rise & Shine! – Formulated to help initiate a natural uplifting.

Meditate & sleep

This will only help in the very early stages of an attack, or when the anxiety is relaxing off. But use relaxation and sleep. This will bring the anxiety under control and get your body used to feeling in a place of calm. The more you feel calm, the longer the anxiety will stay away.

Use film or radio

Distraction can be useful to bring anxiety down, but use relaxation techniques as soon as you feel able. Distraction will bring moments of calm, yes, but it won't bring the long term relief because you need to relax the body and work on the self talk. These are the tools that will make the change.

Take days out

Like meditation, just relaxing all day will also teach you how to cope and deal with the feelings that crop up on a daily routine.

But remember, don't go feeling guilty for looking after yourself. See it as part of the healing journey. Relaxation will allow the nerves to heal and ultimately the anxiety and panic will leave.

Routine

Daily routine is very important when learning to cope with anxiety and panic attacks. I can't emphasize this enough. Meditate at the same times each day, eat at the same times etc. Routine is reassuring to your system and it will allow your body to heal faster. – And remember, allow time to pass. The passage of time with periods of calm will beat this.

Sleep thinking

When you go to bed it's a good idea to change your thinking around to the positive.

Don't think:

'I fear I am going to have a panic attack tonight'

Think:

'I am safe. I am going to sleep well tonight. Tomorrow I will feel better.'

This kind of thinking will gently creep into your subconscious and the fear will go, giving you the confidence you need to not only get through the night, but the day as well.

On waking after a night's sleep

Waking can not only be stressful but can bring on sadness and depression because you tend to think about the day ahead and whether you are going to cope. The best way to help with this is to get up on opening your eyes. Be mindful on your thoughts and concentrate on getting washed and dressed. Thinking ahead panics the mind, so keep it simple, and if physical symptoms do arise, work through them as best you can without attaching too much fear to them. I say too much, because it is very difficult to switch the fear off completely, this is something you will have to learn. Eventually you will find mornings easier, but it helps if you have somewhere to go, or are meeting with someone.

Broken sleep

Broken sleep can come about because panic attacks actually happen during the night and this can be very frightening as we feel more vulnerable than during the daylight hours. Like coping during the day, commit to the following.

○ **Sip water with Rescue Remedy added.**

○ **Try not and let your mind concentrate on the symptoms.**

○ **Keep the reassurance going you are fine, these are only symptoms of anxiety.**

○ **If you can talk with someone reassuring, then do so, this will help calm the panics. Rationalise why you may feel the way you do. Was is because you are overtired?**

Consumed the wrong foods? A particular stress in the day? Bring logic into the fearful situation and this will dissolve the anxiety.

O Distract with a film or radio show.

O Breathe.

O Know this will pass.

O You are safe.

Listen to your body:

O Learn when your body needs to rest.

O Learn what times your body needs food.

O Learn when you need to switch off and relax.

O Get plenty of sleep, this is the time your body heals.

O When you feel you really can't cope in a situation, avoid and try another day.

Learning simple things like the above will put off the feelings of anxiety, eventually eliminating them altogether, because your confidence will grow and your body will become used to a state of calm. The trick here is to be easy on yourself. Resist the self berating, take things easy, and again, remember not to feel guilty for doing so.

Try not to react to the sensation

The sensations are scary. I can't deny that. They are trying to scare you, that is what anxiety does, it puts you in a false belief you are in danger and you could possibly die. But this is untrue, and the sooner you can get a hold on this fact, the sooner you'll cope with this disorder.

After a frightening moment

The worst has happened, you feel steamrollered and your mind is racing on what's wrong and will it happen again. This is fear in its rawest form. Now, and this is the hardest part, you need to reassure yourself everything is fine. You can do this by:

O **Positive self talk.**

O **Talking with somebody positive.**

O **Plenty of rest and time.**

O **Try not dwelling over the feelings because this will only bring them back. <u>Remember, Fear breeds Fear.</u>**

Time is our saviour. Time and rest brings with it peace, which brings confidence in our own bodies not to do the anxiety again. Time is a great healer, and thankfully the human brain is good at forgetting the nitty gritty of pain. The first number of times can be devastating, and the after-effects can last days, weeks, even months, but by practicing these techniques, you will get the after-effects down to minutes, then not at all. It is hard. I am not going to sit here and lie to you, but you do have it in you to beat this. You do. However tired and downtrodden you feel right now, things shall improve, life will get better for you.

Remember, everyday is a new day, don't let the previous days bad experiences define you.

Finally, live in the moment

Regressing back to the past and how your life was better before all this happened isn't going to help. Neither is looking to the future and worrying whether you are ever going to achieve the type of things you want. This creates panic. In our current world, we are told we have to live the dream and get there as fast as possible, otherwise we are some kind of failure. This breeds panic. So it's no wonder we are inflicted with anxiety. We are told constantly time is moving on, you should be at this stage at this particular point in your life. They imply you are a failure if you are alone, don't have a job that pays enough, and don't have numerous friends. This makes us sad and lonely because we feel we aren't normal and we believe there must be something wrong. WE MUST BE NORMAL LIKE EVERYONE ELSE!!! Only, there isn't a normal person on this planet. What is normal?? It just doesn't exist. In truth, we all just cope as best we can.

So:

O Feel the feeling.

O Tell yourself everything is fine, you are safe.

O Talk with somebody. A person saying you are okay can dissipate the feelings.

O Relax as best you can. Keep the internal dialogue going you are safe and you are not going to die.

O Breathe deep, and whatever you do, do not dwell on the sensation.

O Think about what you are doing in the moment. Don't think about the future or picture yourself in pain or dying.

O By repeatedly not reacting to the sensation, you will find the time it affects you will slowly diminish. Where once it made you ill for a whole day and shattered your confidence, with practice it will only last minutes. The more you ignore and tell yourself it's just anxiety, the stronger you will become in not letting these frightening sensations defeat you.

O Watch funny movies or listen to uplifting music.

O Try not to think everyone is having a better life than you, because this is untrue. They have their own problems; they are just very good at hiding them.

O Try not sitting and longing for better times. Think and act on what you can achieve in the moment, however small.

O Have something to eat. Blood sugar levels might have dropped increasing anxiety.

O Self congratulate, no matter how small the success.

A day dealing with anxiety

There is a lot to think about in this chapter, and I know it can not only be overwhelming, but sometimes difficult to remember everything when in a moment of anxiety. So, to make things easier, I am going to plan out a day for you which will bring calm, especially if you make time to do this as often as you can.

O First on waking, sit up and sip some water with Rescue Remedy added, and any other flower remedies you are currently taking.

O Next run a bath and add a calming bubble bath and some aromatherapy oils that promote relaxation. Also add some flower remedies, eg. Rescue Remedy, Chill Out, Rise and Shine mixes. Soak in the bath for twenty minutes to half an hour. (This stage can be done at the end of the day if you prefer).

O Dry off and get dressed. Meditate for twenty minutes with a guided meditation or hypnotherapy **CD**.

O Sip your flower remedies.

O Drink hot water with a slice of lemon and a slice of lime in it. (Brings calm and flushes your stomach of the previous day's food).

O Eat some healthy breakfast.

O Place some aromatherapy oils in an oil burner to promote relaxation.

O Sip your flower remedies every ten to fifteen minutes.

O Call someone and have a chat.

O If your stomach is okay with it, why not have a fresh vegetable green juice. Very high in all the vitamins and minerals your body needs to repair itself. (Search online about how juicing can help with anxiety).

O Watch a funny movie.

O Middle of the day, meditate. (I use an aromatherapy/flower essence spray to prepare the room for meditation and aid relaxation) e.g. 'Aura Cleanse' and 'Energy Balance' sprays available online. www.creaturecomforters.co.uk

O Eat some lunch.

O Hot water and lemon drink.

O Relax and read a book. Do a hobby that doesn't take up much energy. Write your diary.

O Now congratulate yourself on doing so well today and

for coping.

O Eat a well balanced dinner.

O Hot water and lemon/lime drink.

O Meditate again and get an early night.

This a great routine that promotes calm in the mind and body. I am not saying carry this out every day. You will have work, and other daily routines to do. But you will be able to fit many aspects within your day to day tasks. Coping strategies are about working with techniques that calm your body and mind, so you can operate within your daily life, and eventually start to feel the panics release their hold on you. It all starts with a single step. If you can only do one thing on the list today, then so be it. That is good enough right now, tomorrow or next week you might be able to do two things, and so on. Every little victory is one step closer to your goal in beating this. Be happy with yourself for trying this, you are making positive steps and that has to be celebrated in itself. You can do this, I know you can. Anxiety is tricking you to be unwell, but you are stronger than anxiety, you will get through what seems intolerable right now and I am here to help.

Last coping strategy

So you see not one thing will eliminate your anxiety, but all aspects teach your mind and body to stay calm and not hit the emergency button. It's not easy, and it takes time and practice to master coping strategies, but the more you can ride the sensations and work out what times of the day they are likely to strike, you can put in coping strategies to deal with them. Which leads me nicely onto the panic diary.

The panic diary

Simply, write down what times the anxiety attacks happen every day for the next few weeks. Date the day and write the time you found the attack or feeling of unwellness struck. It's that easy.

The purpose of all this is to track and see if there is a pattern emerging. Say panic always strikes at mid morning. Would it benefit eating something at this time? Or would it be beneficial to meditate before the feelings start? This way you can train your body to break the pattern and eliminate the anxiety from this particular part of the day. Maybe just before bedtime you become anxious because you see bedtime as a frightening time as panic has always struck during the night. Write your thoughts down, meditate, take Rescue Remedy, and try and change your thinking from fear based to positive. Again, this won't happen and fix the problem over night, but the more times you do this, you will slowly get a hold on anxiety and your confidence will return once more.

'You are doing incredibly well, so please be proud of your achievements, you are far stronger than this disorder is leading you to believe.'

Summary

Tick

Box

☐Use the coping strategies to calm the panic.

☐Allow time to pass and don't give up, you will get through this.

☐Allow the feelings to pass without attaching the fear

---

to them. Although this can be hard at first, you will overtime get the hang of this.

☐Normality doesn't exist. Don't aspire to be 'NORMAL.' Different is far more interesting.

☐Don't allow society to dictate how you should be. You are in the right place you are meant to be at this given moment.

☐Keep a panic diary so you can track when anxiety strikes. By doing this you can adjust your coping strategies to warn off impending attacks.

☐Don't think you are of less value than anyone else. You are stronger than you realise.

☐Remember, 'YOU ARE SAFE.'

- 18 -

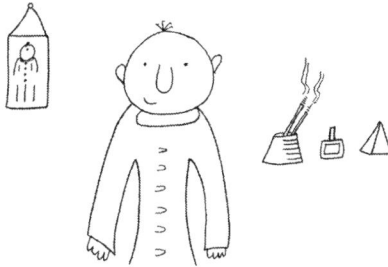

Energy Healing

Positive healing for the mind body & spirit

I think you will be pleasantly surprised by what this old form of therapy can do for you concerning anxiety and panic attacks. It's powerful, and it can affect you on many levels, i.e. mind body and spirit. But it can also re-teach your body to know what it feels like to be in a state of relaxation, instead of full blown anxiety. Even if it is only for an hour, you will see the symptoms subside and enjoy a period of time feeling better in yourself. And like everything here, repetition brings with it results.

Periods of Calm = Less Anxiety and Anxiety Symptoms

In our daily lives we don't get the down time to relax, I mean really relax to the point you are unaware of your body. Quality relaxation where the mind and body switch off and your batteries have the opportunity to recharge. – Healing allows you to do this. It allows for your entire system to experience such a state of deep relaxation, where your mind can shut down and all the pains will melt away. A place of total bliss.

Healing can feel like dropping all the heavy bags to the floor and flopping on the sofa after a busy day. A relief for you mentally and physically from the constant roller coaster ride that anxiety can bring. And in the beginning, even if this feeling of calm only lasts for a short period, it's got to be worth it. As any anxiety sufferer will gladly tell you, they just want to get off the ride of fear, however long that may be.

The basics

It's widely believed we are energy beings, and that our bodies contain channels called meridians which act like the super highway for our energy to flow. These are connected via the seven energy centres aligned down the spine called chakras (a Sanskrit word for 'wheel') that absorb and emit life force. Each chakra governs a particular area of the body with specific emotional issues.

They consist of:

Crown chakra – (Violet) Top of head. Spirituality, higher consciousness, Union with higher self.

Brow chakra – (Indigo) Third eye. Intuition, imagination, insight, clairvoyance, concentration.

Throat chakra – (Sky blue) Adams apple. Communication, creative expression, soul realisation.

Heart – (Green) Centre of chest. Compassion, forgiveness, understanding, unconditional love.

Solar plexus – (Yellow) 5- 7cm above navel. Intellect, personal power, will, confidence.

Sacral – (Orange) Navel area. Gut instincts, emotions, vitality.

Root – (Red) Base of spine. Grounding, stability, courage, perseverance.

The chakras and their positioning

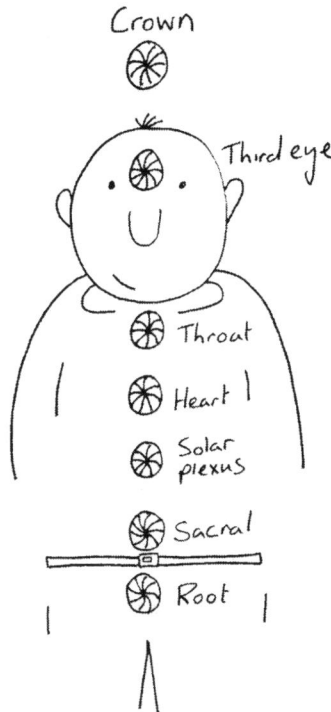

Where the free flow of energy throughout our chakras indicate well being, ill heath indicates a blockage or imbalance has occurred, and we need some treatment to rectify this. It can be caused by drugs, bad nutrition, injury, and mental / emotional issues such as shock, grief, or negative thinking. This is why it's so important to stand tall, sit upright, and allow the free flow of energy to pass through the entire system. And not slump, like we all do when in pain. It's natural. A small child, and even us as adults, will take the foetal position when ill. That's not a criticism, but when we are restricted in this way, we tend to experience congestion in our entire energy system, only adding to the pain physically and on an emotional level as well.

But it hurts?

The reason being your energy is squeezing through restricted channels. Think of it like someone standing on a hose pipe and reducing the flow of water. When that person steps off however, flow is resumed. By straightening your body the pains shall be there for a small amount of time, but soon they'll disappear and you will feel much better in yourself. Not to mention a little bit taller!

Understanding what energy feels like

Because this is likely to be a bit new I'd like you to carry out the following exercise. By feeling your own life energy, this will give you a better understanding with what you are working with here. Energy healing is an incredibly powerful tool in your quest to beating anxiety and panic attacks, and even though you might have disregarded it in the past, I strongly urge you to consider checking this out.

Rugby ball exercise

'Stand tall and raise your arms so they are resting straight in front of you. Now I want you to imagine you're holding a rugby ball. Palms facing each other, fingers pointing upwards, a rugby ball width apart. Good. Start moving your arms in position directly up and down.'

(see picture).

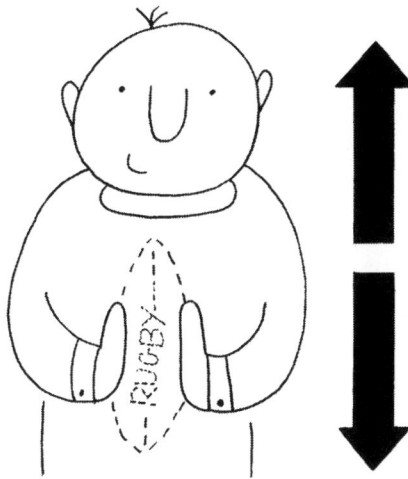

Rugby ball exercise/feeling your own energy

After a few movements you will begin to feel your life energy. Tingling in the palms of your hands and maybe some heat mixed in there as well.

It's amazing, but that's you, the very energy of who you are, and who you are going to be in the future.

Healing the pain

Through my own journey, I decided to take up healing so I could help others heal their own life pains. And it never ceases to amaze me how powerful balancing the chakras really is. I've worked on clients so hunched over and bearing the weight of the world, only for them to jump off my healing bed more confident and willing to get better. Which is why rebalancing is so highly important. Just like understanding the parts of our lives that put us out of balance, and then make the changes so our energy centres remain rotating at the correct speed and shining bright. The rubbish that life throws at us clog the chakras, and they become drab and sluggish. By cleaning them, we feel light, confident, and willing to reach our desires.

Chakras in more detail

Crown chakra

Normal – Magnetic personality, achieves miracles, transcendent, and feels generally at peace with everything in life.

Blocked - **(Chakra spins sluggishly or not at all)** Feel constantly exhausted, can't make decisions, a sense of not belonging.

Too open – **(Chakra spins too fast)** Psychotic or manic depressive. Confused sexual expression. Frustrated with a sense of unrealised power.

Third eye

When blocked the sufferer experiences a whirling imagination. May fear the worst could happen, creating headaches, and a feeling of memory constipation. (Stuffy head).

Too open – Dogmatic, authoritarian, arrogant, highly logical.

Blocked – Has a deep fear of success, sets sights too low, undisciplined.

Balanced – Highly intuitive, not attached to material things, charismatic, might experience strange phenomena.

Throat

The throat is your communication point, but this becomes suppressed when anxiety is present. Remember how hard it was to speak during an attack? And now, explaining how you feel? Anger and frustration further closes this chakra. May suffer a sore throat through lack of expression. Wants to say 'No,' but says 'Yes' anyway.

Normal – Communicator with strong confident voice. Speaks their feelings and has little problem talking in various situations.

Blocked - Causes tightness in throat and trouble speaking, especially in front of a group. Finds the need to clear throat regularly. Cause can be down to childhood traumas, e.g. told regularly to shut up, spoken over, made to feel comments are worthless. - In order to deal with rejection, words are suppressed, making the person choose to neglect responsibility for growing up and taking charge of life.

Heart

Normal -The heart is for love and harmony for oneself and those around.

Blocked - Instead we feel pains in the chest as the love we feel for ones self and others has gone. Opening up this chakra after a period of shutting out through fear of more hurt, may be uncomfortable. This should not be confused with a heart attack. The discomfort is one of emotion not physicality.

This is not an indication you don't care, but have become afraid of letting love in while expressing love for others. Ridicule and rejection, leading to fear, are key areas which cause the clamping down of this chakra.

Solar plexus

Sensitivity to situations. The centre for human recognition and self worth; also where unresolved situations create stress.

Normal - Once the solar plexus has been strengthened and stimulated it gives you true inner power. You'll be able to shrug off criticism, fears of rejection, and release all worries from standing apart from the crowd. Also a sense of self respect and the ability to handle any situation.

Blocked – **(Chakra spins sluggishly or not at all)** overly concerned about what others think, insecure, fearful of being alone. Needs constant reassurance.

Spins too fast – Angry; tends to be a workaholic and very judgmental. Shows signs of being controlling and superior over others.

Sacral

Normal – Trusting, expressive and attuned to own feelings. Creative.

Blocked – **(Chakra spins sluggishly or not at all)** overly sensitive, hard on themselves, and feels guilty for no reason. Frigid or impotent.

Spins too fast – Emotionally unbalanced, a fantasist, manipulative and sexually addictive.

Root

Normal – Demonstrates self mastery, high physical energy, grounded, and health.

Blocked – **(Chakra spins sluggishly or not at all)** emotionally needy, low self esteem, self destructive behaviour, and fearful.

Spins too fast – Bullying, overly materialistic, self-centered and engages in physical foolhardiness.

How to balance the chakras

Meditations and crystals are a great way to balance all your chakras, books and CD's are available aiding you to do this. I found 'Chakra Clearing' by Doreen Virtue (CD and Tape) excellent for this. Readily available from Amazon. Book with CD version ISBN (1-4019-0277-4) Also available for digital download.

Be healed by another person

Although the books and CDs are highly effective, I'd recommend having a healer work on you from the outset. An experienced healer is worth their weight in gold, and you'll feel the benefits much quicker this way.

Note: The thing to remember when coming out of any healing or meditation, is to take a few minutes out. Sitting still while you can regroup. Any sudden movements might cause a strong feeling of giddiness and is best avoided. *'Drink plenty of water.'*

Also: Just breathe naturally. Enjoy the moment of calm before resuming your normal daily life.

Tiredness is not uncommon either, so a cat nap in the day rejuvenates the soul and your very being.

Some types of healing

Reiki

One method of healing is Reiki, the Japanese word for life energy. A form of powerful healing known to tap the unseen flow of energy that permeates every living thing. Reiki, believed to originate from a branch of Tibetan Buddhism, was traditionally passed down from master to student, but this nearly became its downfall.

As time progressed, this ancient art became lost only to be rediscovered by a Japanese minister, Dr. Mikao Usui, around the 19th century. Believing he could truly find the answer to Reiki once more, he travelled up a mountain side and meditated for several days until the very thing he sought appeared. Four symbols. Once these symbols were attuned by any student, the power of Reiki could be unleashed.

Since then, Reiki is practiced all over the world, but because of the attuning process involved, healing will need to be conducted by someone who has been attuned already.

Quantum Touch

Founder Richard Gordon.

Some say this is like Reiki on steroids. And using it myself I'd say I'd have to agree. QT work has the ability to move bones, sort emotional issues and even heal cancer. It's powerful and highly recommended. I have used QT to successfully heal panic and anxiety a number of times now and I wouldn't be without it.

Tip*: 'For more information visit: www.quantumtouch.com. Check out their 'Five colour meditation.' Excellent CD for balancing the body on all levels.'*

Reflexology

This is a very old therapy. Thousands of years ago Eastern Healers used pressure on parts of the foot which corresponded with an area, or particular organ in the body. For example, the toes being the head and brain, the heel representing the pelvic area. And where there are two organs, such as the kidneys, the reflexologist will work on the left foot for the left kidney, and the right foot for the right kidney, and so on. Discomfort from the patient shows up where a blockage is present and will need freeing for the energy to flow once more. Chakras are also worked on by some, giving the patient not only physical healing but mental as well.

Aromatherapy

By using natural oils of plants and flowers, an experienced aromatherapist can heal, beautify, and boost emotional and spiritual well being. It's said the oils pass through the skin and enter the bloodstream where it's carried around the body. Another view says these oils contain the universal life force energy of the plant, which interacts with our own life energy to stimulate, subdue, or balance our seven chakras.

Once experienced, you might feel tired but notice a gentle calmness about you, which is why it's so good for ridding anxiety that's been causing stress lately. But please note, as with all these therapies, go regularly. It will bring your body more in line with where it should be, slowly diminishing the pains and sickness created by the adrenaline.

Spiritual

This is a very powerful way of healing, and when conducted in the right manner, can bring amazing results. Sometimes referred to as energy work, the healer unblocks energy around the client's body bringing calm on a physical and mental level.

Energy is called from the divine (universal energy) along with healing guides and angelic helpers who assist in the healing process. A session will typically last one hour but there is no limit on the number of sessions you have. I recommend at least once every fortnight, but weekly is ideal.

Jin-Shin

Jin Shin, otherwise known as Jin Shin Jyutsu, is a non intrusive healing where the healer places their hands on the patient's body in a particular way to promote energy flow. It's not too dissimilar to acupuncture, except in this case, there are no needles.

See *'Survival Kit'* for a couple of exercises. But you might like to search out a practitioner for some full sessions.

EFT

EFT, or Emotional Freedom Technique, is a very clever way of releasing energy blocks within your system by the simple use of tapping and affirmations. This is something you can read up on and practice yourself in the privacy of your own home. But the great thing with this type of healing is, you can also use it discreetly when you're out and about, and it takes less than a minute to do. This simple, highly effective technique, works by removing limiting negative emotions in your life and in doing so, helps takeaway the body tensions and sensations you may be feeling right now.

I recommend the book:

Enjoy Emotional Freedom by Steve Wells and Dr David Lake.

OHB – Optimum Health Balance

Optimum Health Balance is a holistic system of kinesiology used to balance the whole energy system of the body and to therefore help achieve, physical, emotional, mental and spiritual balance. Energy is generally channelled through the hands of the practitioner through a healing icon placed on the body or in the energy field above it.

Others

There are many other types of therapies out there, some you will find and use because a therapist has a particular liking for them and thinks they will be beneficial. But whichever one you use, just lie back, take a deep breath, and let somebody rub, prod, hold, or pass healing energy from above. - Whichever techniques work for you, enjoy.

Note: *'Visit an alternative health shop where they will be able to assist you in all your healing requirements.'*

Summary

Tick

Box

☐We are energy, when something becomes blocked we fall ill.

☐We have seven main energy centres called chakras.

☐Stand & sit upright, this allows the energy to flow freely and relieves pain.

☐By working on the chakras, we can regain balance physically and mentally.

☐Have a fully qualified healer do it for you.

☐Healing should not be seen as an alternative to prescribed drugs but a complimentary therapy.

☐Try a chakra healing CD. Doreen Virtue 'Chakra Clearing'(Amazon) or 'The Five Colour Meditation.' (www.quantumtouch.com).

☐Healing is safe.

☐Healing is deeply calming for a busy mind and tired body.

☐Find a practitioner in your area who will be able to assist you.

☐Relax and enjoy the experience.

☐Remember, 'YOU ARE SAFE.'

- 19 -

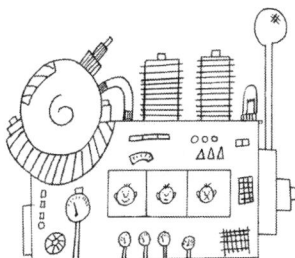

Our Emotion Engine

Inside us all we have an emotion engine. It's a complex device that's not always understood. Here I'm going to shed some light on why you can feel the way you do.

The two basic emotions in life – <u>Love</u> and <u>Fear</u>

Surprisingly, we only have two emotions, love and fear. All our other emotions are variations of these. For example:

Anxiety	*Guilt*
Anger	*Hurt*
Control	*Loneliness*
Confusion	*Sadness*
Depression	*Shame*

These are all fear based emotions, where the following are love based emotions:

Compassion	*Joy*
Contentment	*Satisfaction*
Caring	*Trust*

Happiness   *Truth*

All these can come in varying degrees of intensity, some mild, others moderate, and finally full blown. For instance, anger in a mild form can be felt as disgust or dismay, move it on a stage further, and you feel offended or exasperated. Again, at its peak comes hate and rage. The emotion that underpins anger is always **Fear.**

You can control your emotions

In daily life, we see somebody who seemingly functions normally, only to suddenly explode in a fit of anger at something that seems pretty trivial to everybody else around. This is a sign this person has repressed their emotions. But however hard they try, from time to time it leaks out. And so the more a person tries to control their emotions, the more they resist control, and thus, the person becomes increasingly frightened of what's seen as 'loss of emotional control'. It's another vicious circle.

In today's world we are taught to suppress our emotions, it's seen as some kind of weakness to show how we are actually feeling, which buries them deeper within us where they can make us unwell. Instead we should learn how to recognise them, turn them around, and of course release them in a safe manner. Suppressed emotions are the primary cause of panic attacks. The more we suppress, the more out of control our emotions become.

✌☺Bach flower remedy to take:

Take Cherry Plum found in Rescue Remedy. (Counteracts fear of losing mind. - Irrational thoughts or behavior. Brings mental calm).

Core issues and emotions

Many of us suffer from emotions caused by core issues. They come about because of family patterns, or patterns that we have created for ourselves. As an example, you keep falling for the wrong type of partner time and time again. The same with friends, who repeatedly don't turn out to be the person you thought they were. Then you wonder, 'what have I done to deserve all this, I'm not a bad person am I?' - No you're not. You just need to recognise where the problem lies and re-address it.

Some examples of core issues are:

O**Lack of confidence.**

O**Fear of not fitting in.**

O**Low self esteem.**

O**Self sabotage.**

O**Emotional or physical abuse.**

O**Trying to live up to other people's expectations.**

O**Too higher standards.**

O**Trying to please everyone all of the time.**

O**Unable to say 'No' and honour yourself instead.**

By gently working through your emotions with the aid of the flower remedies, you'll soon identify the core issues that need resolving. For instance, one of my core issues was taking on board other people's negative opinions of me. I repeatedly came into contact with the kind of people that thought I was their personal door mat. By standing up for myself and being more assertive, and showing them they couldn't treat me that way anymore, made that particular core issue become resolved.

Emotional abuse

You might think emotional abuse is the poor cousin to physical abuse, but in fact, it is just as serious and harming. The mind can become severely traumatized through continual abuse, and instead of walking away, you take the abuse and feel there is no way out. Sometimes you might even think you deserve it, or are afraid of rocking the boat. But what's happening is, their opinion of you is slowly becoming your reality.

Abuse can come in the following ways:

Degrading   Humiliating   Insulting   Rejection

Isolating   Ridiculing   Terrorizing   Silent treatment

Denial of emotional response

Nobody on this planet should suffer this, or any other kind of abuse for that matter. And if you are in a situation with this going on, however hard it might be, get help, you deserve the very best.

'Finding someone trusted to talk to, and admitting you have a problem, is the first step towards healing the situation.'

ʮ@Flower remedies to take: Agrimony, Centuary and Larch.

Afraid to feel

It's sad, but more and more people are afraid to really express their feelings. This comes about because we are led to believe we can't show our emotions, and we are afraid of what others will think of us if we do.

In this scenario, the more we suppress our emotions, the more unwell we become. So, feel, release, and enjoy a life of fulfillment and serenity.

> **ꝰ⊛Flower remedy to take is: Agrimony**

Identifying repressed emotions

When something happens and we feel it's too difficult or painful to cope with, we often get busy, exercise more, drink or eat more, or just pretend it never actually happened in the first place. As a result the emotions get stuck in our bodies contributing to hypertension, stomach disorders, and a general feeling of being unwell.

To release we must bring that emotion up, feel that emotion, and gently let it go.

Methods people use to avoid feeling their emotions:

O Any type of compulsive behaviour.

O Ignoring the feelings.

O Always keeping busy so not to feel.

O Working excessively.

O Burying angry emotions under peace.

O Extreme mood swings.

O Keeping conversations superficial.

O Pretending it never happened.

Not surprisingly, it takes a heck of a lot of energy to keep emotions suppressed, that's why fatigue and depression are major factors here. The next list shows some symptoms that come about because of buried emotions.

○ Low self esteem.

○ Lack of confidence.

○ Laughing on the outside but really crying within.

○ Withdrawn.

○ Difficulty in accepting yourself and others.

○ Pretending something hasn't upset you when actually it has.

○ Feeling anger some time after the event.

○ Rarely talking about feelings.

○ Difficulty in talking about yourself.

○ A tightness in the stomach or a knot in the throat.

○ A lack of ambition or motivation.

Identifying buried or repressed emotions

Sleep diary - The sleep diary can be added as an extra to your normal day to day diary. By writing down your night time dreams, you can identify what is going on in your mind. Do this for a number of months, and patterns will emerge, identifying which emotions need to be addressed. Often the emotions you feel in your dreams are the very ones that you are repressing and burying inside.

Little and unimportant hurts – Write down all the things that you've dismissed as very unimportant, or don't matter, when deep inside they matter a great deal. Like the kids walking in with dirty shoes on a new carpet, or the washing up left on the front room table for the umpteenth time. Situations you've buried within because you don't want any conflict, but really they have a lasting effect on you.

By writing, it helps you identify what's causing your mixed emotions, and brings things back into perspective so you can deal with them more easily. Even if that means finding an agreeable resolution between both parties.

Repressed emotions example - A young woman can't understand whenever her partner leaves for a business trip, she feels abandoned and nervous inside. The root cause actually goes back to her childhood when her parents' marriage split up. The feeling she felt then, and buried when seeing her father leave, still have large repercussions today.

Understanding why and talking about this, allowed her to finally feel the emotions and release the blockage. Writing about it can evoke the repressed emotions and allow a successful release.

ᘰ❁ **Flower remedies to take: Agrimony, Aspen, Chicory, and Mimulus.**

What makes you really angry? – Write down what really gets on your wick, the things that wind you up so tight you feel you'll literally explode. And it doesn't have to be just people related, it might be the weather, an object you use daily, or perhaps the traffic on the way to work. Whatever and whoever, write it down, and get that anger out of your system where it can be aired.

ᘰ❁ **Remedies to take: Agrimony, Willow, Holly, Mustard, and Beech.**

Don't forget the positive – Remember, after all that negative scribbling, write down all the positives about yourself. If you don't do this, you will end up with an unrealistic picture of yourself, because in reality, you are probably a caring loving compassionate human being. So remind yourself of this constantly. See the good, concentrate on the good, feel the good.

'As powerful as writing down your emotions is, the power of releasing can be greatly increased by talking it over with a trusted friend, counsellor, or anybody else who can guarantee full confidentiality.' - (Very important for the mind).

The art of releasing emotions

Emotions are neither good or bad, they are there not to be fought, so don't block, fight, or run away from them. Instead feel them and slowly they'll dissipate and normal health can be resumed.

The response – Firstly, it's not a good idea to identify the emotion and go straight into a release like a bull in a china shop. This is a time to sit back and think, and ask yourself, 'what would be the ideal way of dealing with it?'

I say this, because the situation might mean losing your job, a close family member, or even your marriage. That is why I say proceed with caution here, especially before going and saying something you wished you hadn't.

So the kind of questions you should ask yourself are:

O **Are you being true to yourself?**

O **Is a direct approach the right way to proceed?**

O **What would be the consequences if I dealt directly with the person/situation?**

222

○ Will I be able to talk to this person?

○ Can I talk without venting my anger?

○ Am I reacting to this situation, or is it in fact connected to a past event?

○ What do I expect from this discussion?

○ Are my expectations realistic?

○ Should I discuss it with a trusted friend before proceeding?

These questions will tell you if you're ready to do this in the now, and the best approach. Keeping things as calm as possible is advantageous, because two or more angry people can just make the whole situation far worse than it need be.

'Try: writing a letter. Say everything you'd like to say, and if some things are a bit on the strong side, take it out. You can either rehearse it over in your head before speaking to the person, or hand them your letter.'

Warning! If you are at the rage stage, some of this anger needs to be vented beforehand. Because rage is a volatile animal at best, and uncontrollable actions can result which will probably be regretted later.

A good punch and shout can make all the difference – This is more related to anger and hurt, but physically, doing something can be beneficial. And just before you pick up the boxing gloves and walk out the door fuming, I am not talking about harm to another person. No matter how angry you are with them, that just makes matters worse. I'm talking about venting in safety.

Methods of release:

1. Go into an empty room, or take a drive somewhere and scream as loudly as you can. Allow yourself to cry your feeling.

2. Take a pillow and hit it. Feel the pain inside every time you hit that pillow.

3. Write down all your hurts, your anger, how fearful you really are. And write what's been going through your mind today and how you feel about It. - Feel the feeling, don't be afraid of it.

Remember in any situation or discussion:

Anger evokes Anger   *Calm evokes Calm*

Compassion evokes Compassion

Whatever method you employ, it's important to acknowledge it's alright to have feelings of anger, hurt or rage, and this is a safe way to accept your feelings. So often we are afraid to lose control, or feel the sheer intensity that's within us. Yet the more you choose to ignore these feelings, the bigger they become.

When releasing it's important to remember these points:

○ **Recognise the emotion you are feeling for what it is. Anger, hate, rage.**

○ **Concentrate on the emotion, say 'I am angry.'**

○ **Don't be afraid to accept your feelings. Working through your feelings helps take away some of the power they have over you.**

🌿 Flower remedies to take: Agrimony, Willow, Holly, and Mustard.

Speak the truth – As hard as it might feel to begin with, start to feel more comfortable when talking about yourself with a trusted friend. Go deep within, say how you feel, say how a situation affects you today in the greatest of detail.

We commonly hide things inside of us because we are ashamed, or perceive ourselves as a bad person, yet by telling your story, it helps get a good perspective on the whole situation. Yet keep it singular. Tell one person and don't keep repeating the same story over and over. If this happens, it turns into resentment, (reoccurring negative thinking), and that's another problem. – Otherwise write down what's in your head.

Resentments – This is a reoccurring anger which goes around your head time and time again, thinking about someone who has upset you. This is unhelpful, making you feel agitated inside, yet has no effect on the person who hurt you. – Realise you can't change that person, but you can learn to accept them as they are, forgive them, and move on with your life.

Letting go

Take a piece of paper and put the person's name at the very top. And start with the following;

I WISH ……….. THE MOST WONDERFUL LIFE IN THE WORLD. I WISH THEM ALL THE LUCK ON OFFER AND THAT ALL THEIR DREAMS MAY COME TRUE. I FORGIVE HIM/HER FOR THE HURT HE/SHE HAS CAUSED, AND SO I HOLD NO GRUDGE AGAINST HIM/HER.

Now list all their positive attributes, and by doing this, a shift will occur within you and bring with it peace of mind. Remember, it may take time though.

Note: *'It takes great strength and courage to forgive and move on.'*

Although it's important to honour an injustice has taken place, it's equally important to recognise your own behaviour and accept responsibility for your own actions. *'When you do this, the emotions around a situation lose their hold upon you.'*

Remember – *'It's not just what happens to us that makes a difference. It's how we choose to either react or respond to it.'*

Step back from the situation – When your emotions are high and you find it difficult to reduce the intensity of them, step back. If somebody snaps at you, or are short in their words, it might be because they are still living their particular problem in their own mind, and you just got caught up in it. Realising this, it can be easier to release the emotions and just put it down to bad timing. *'Don't take it personally.'*

Acknowledge your fears – It's not always easy to admit you have fears, but by doing this, it also helps release your emotions.

Are you afraid of?

Being alone	*Ridicule*	*Losing prestige*
Abandonment	*Lack of money*	*The unknown*
Loneliness	*Adventure*	*Death*
Losing somebody	*Going crazy*	*Suffering*
Losing face	*Lack of love*	*Self Worth*

Fears are tricky for anyone. Some you can ignore and get along fine, like a fear of spiders; and others you can act as if you are unafraid. But as you become aware of your own fears, you'll notice some will come and go without much doing on your part. It might be a thought in your head, a slight change in attitude, but if you don't allow the fear to stop you, you can move forward in greater confidence.

Take care – Taking care of, and honouring yourself is the biggest way you can feel self love and gain self respect. Don't punish yourself for your actions, be gentle on yourself, understand why, and how you can remedy the problem. After all, you are human, and like all of us, you've been born with a full set of emotions that are hard to live with at times. But with time patience and practice, you can learn how to deal with situations, people, and more importantly yourself more effectively.

Understanding yourself is a big step forward

Forgiveness – By the act of forgiving yourself and others who have caused you hurt, it will bring a feeling of inner peace, and with this newfound peace a sense of being more in control. It's not always easy to forgive and forget, but with time and a strong direction in life, the hurts will gradually seem less important than they once were.

Overall – You don't have to put up with situations that bring conflict and upsets, or the kind of people that you can't plainly get along with. And I guess, at the end of the day it's all down to experience. Knowing when to fight and stand your ground, or walk away. Only you can decide this.

'Realise the things you can change and accept the things you cannot.'

'Remember, __FAITH__ cancels out __FEAR__, you can't have both

together.'

Faith – Fear = Achievement + Confidence

Summary

Tick

Box

☐There are only two basic emotions, _Love_ & _Fear._ Any other emotion is a variation of these.

☐You can learn to control your emotions.

☐In the modern world we are often taught to suppress our emotions which can make us feel unwell. Instead, recognise and release them in a safe manner.

☐Don't be afraid to show emotion. You are not weak when you do so.

☐Use writing as a way of identifying suppressed emotions and bringing them back into perspective.

☐Always replace negative with positive. Realise all the good qualities about yourself and repeatedly remind yourself of them.

☐Go hit a pillow if need be. Shout and scream. Get it out of your system.

☐In any situation, anger evokes anger, calm evokes calm. - Flower remedies will be of help here.

☐'YOU ARE SAFE.'

How do you eat an elephant?

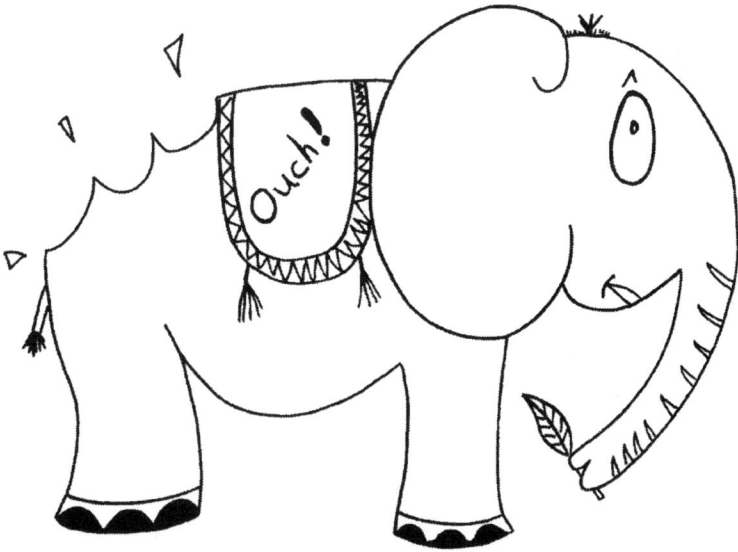

One bite at a time of course

When you look at something, you will find it easier if you take small chunks and deal with them individually, instead of trying to tackle the whole picture in one go.

- 20 -

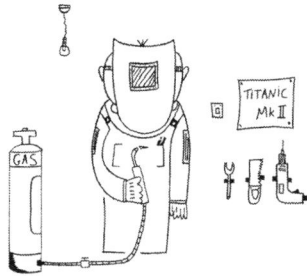

The Beginning of Great Things

Before doing the next exercise, I can say hand on heart this made a big difference. When your mind's racing away every waking minute, these thoughts have effects upon your body. They twist you in knots so tight you reach despair. For me, I wanted to cry, but couldn't. I wanted to end it all straight away, but that wasn't going to happen either. And when a hot drink and a good night's sleep did little to comfort me, I soon came to realise I needed to search for something stronger.

Scared, and very tired, I switched on my faithful laptop unsure to where the coming journey would take me. By emptying all my thinking onto paper, it brought calmness of mind, and a better perspective on why I felt so confused.

And this is where I want to take you right now, by tackling the small things in the here and now, it will help you understand the process of releasing the past and moving forward.

> **This part of the healing programme is extremely powerful; today will be a major step forward for you.**

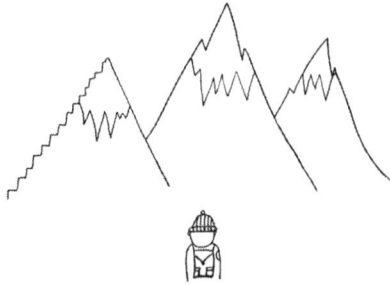

First things first — Small steps BIG STEPS

Starting off, I want you to write down how you feel while reading this. In this moment. Exactly what you think about yourself and the world around you.

Although this might seem like a small step, in reality it's a big step. Admitting how you feel can be emotionally hard, but one we must take, before going up the mountain and conquering the summit of success. Taking this on now would be near impossible, just like a climber wouldn't take on a mountain he'd never trained for. You are going to start on a smaller scale, and when the time comes to tackle the big one, you will be able to do it without a problem.

So for now, try not to hold back, if you feel strongly about something, make sure your voice is heard in the writing. Rant, if you want to rant. Swear if you want to swear, say things that you've been dying to say but felt you couldn't. This is the opportunity to really get what's been bugging you shot clean out of the system.

If you want to tell yourself how pathetic you feel, say so, if you want to tell yourself where you'd like to be, and not where you presently are, say that as well. This is not the time for pussy footing about, ***say what you mean.***

And when you're done, remember to congratulate yourself on a job well done. Not many people have the courage to do this, but you have, you can get all the problems in your mind out today. – If someone made you mad today, yet you walked away saying nothing, write it here. Write whatever you feel you need to write. That's the only rule.

'As an example, I've included the first piece I ever wrote. It's genuine, and I haven't edited its form from the day it was written. Therefore it should serve as a good pointer in the direction you need to take for maximum benefit.'

BIG PROBLEMS

It's just after three in the morning, Monday 2nd of June 2003. I awake to pains in the body, sharp pains accompanied with tiredness, yet I can't sleep.

My brain churns with the 'BIG PROBLEM', or maybe problems. What people have said, what they still say, and this only supports the 'PROBLEM' strengthening it further. Accompany this with an inner drive, to be somebody who stands out from Mr. Average who does the nine to five job. Complains of crap pay, does nothing about it, and forty years later has still not found satisfaction, because they hadn't achieved the very thing that would make them feel like they contributed to society as a whole.

I suppose that inner satisfaction that success brings, whether how small, it's there for other people to see and appreciate.

From school, the drive was there for me but never supported.

Put downs seem to have made it harder. And yes, teachers were a problem. Later an employer, then customers who regularly even

---

today say, 'is this what you really do? - Wash cars?' Their face is one of disbelief, and I must say it is the girls who do it most.

Of course I tell them how busy I am, but the damage is done. I take it on board yet again. Not that I want to. It just happens. Just like when people used to say I don't say much, I'm shy, ugly. Richards being Richard. Wet. This again creates a problem.

Talking, being out and about, all very much feel like an ordeal and has an adverse effect on me.

Sometimes I suffer from tight throat syndrome, so tight in fact I almost puke in the street. Tension does this, and thinking if there is something wrong with me.

Mentally I feel messed up at times, I see people in the standard relationship house thing and then look where I am. Nowhere. Skint and nowhere.

I'm twenty seven, people can't believe it when I say it. Shocked even. That makes me feel a retard in the social stakes, why am I not like other people??? Goes through my head with regularity.

I feel like I'm fighting just to stay alive here, it's tiring, scary as hell, depressing.

But at least keeping busy turns my mind off this for the majority of the time, if it didn't, I'd probably be in even bigger problems.

But then there's the other side of the coin, the inner drive I spoke about. My drive to prove I can do it. To show I'm not thick, finish what I have started and say I escaped the usual rat race and found the inner satisfaction from producing something solid, an experience everybody can enjoy. The novel. Then perhaps an invention to blow the world in energy terms. Show what many inventors have been trying to do for years, but live in fear of losing their lives because of their ideas. I mean who would risk bumping off an internationally acclaimed author? – Am I aiming too high?

If there is one ability I have, that is to learn by discovering what's out there. Tutors/ teachers in the past weren't exactly all that, they never taught me anything new, just past. I couldn't, and still don't see the point why I had to endure the boredom of school.

If you want to really learn, go do it. Yes mistakes will be made, but the work will be all the better for it. I was a remedial student at school, couldn't spell. Couldn't construct sentences. But now when I think back I always wanted to write a novel. This is self taught, practice and reading did this. But I still feel thick, maybe the finished article will dispel this thought, except whatever I do it's not good enough, the old programming finds a way in here too. The constant criticisms.

Yes I want to stick a finger up at how people say I should live. Why do I have to conform to the norm? Who wrote the law we should all be the same anyhow?

But this sickness slows me, sometimes stops me. Concentration can be difficult when staying alive occupies the majority of it. A strong feeling I don't belong. Is this from my mother's theory my father not really wanting to have kids in the first place? I don't know. Maybe.

And so I struggle on. Waking, worrying about age, death. What's going to happen in the future. - Like I said, BIG PROBLEMS.

See how destructive that was? But then if it wasn't, I wouldn't have been in the kind of state I found myself in. The self berating was strong, but I found with more confidence in writing, this kind of material brought with it the ability to really get things off my chest. – A release, a way of venting how I actually felt, instead of masking all the time with a happy face.

It's not a process to fear however, but remember this, sometimes it will hurt. What you're doing is writing how you currently perceive yourself, which equals up to all the years of negative thinking in one tight nit bundle. But you want out, you want all that on paper so you can emerge free from all those destructive thoughts, and feel lighter in yourself.

The exercise. - *'Take a clean sheet of paper and a pen. Sit quietly on your own and write down how you currently feel, and whatever grieves you. It can be as long or short as you like.'*

Once written

By now you should have a piece of writing in front of you, and it's my guess you're probably feeling pretty bashed about, so file it away and take a well earned rest. You've done really well, you've said things that needed to be said, and although it might feel as though nothing's happened, you'll soon come to recognise exactly how this exercise has helped later on in the healing programme.

Positive – day by day

So we have some negativity out of the way; now we want some positive to take its place. You've just seen how destructive thoughts can affect us, but what if we'd started life in the positive and continued? We'd be so positive, in fact, there would be nothing stopping us from whatever our dreams desire. And yes, just because we came off track a bit in the past, from today, there's no reason why we can't put it right.

Here is my positive version of what I showed you before.

NO PROBLEMS

I can understand the pains in my body are not anything to worry about, they are a result of the fight or flight response. I'm not going to die. It's scary yes, but I can overcome this, I will not lie down and give up. - No way.

Sure people have said some things that affected me in the past, but who cares? I don't. I'm me now, not what somebody else thinks I should be. It takes courage to stand out from the crowd, make a difference, strive for the dream. This is a gift not a defect.

The rat race is something to be avoided at all costs, surviving outside and dodging the grappling hook is worth it. No matter who tries to drag me in kicking and screaming, I fight back, I make self employment work because deep within I know the nine to five job would be my downfall. It would be my new nightmare.

Yes people might laugh, say things to make me look stupid. But hang on, who's the stupid one here? The person who has control of his life, or the one who is controlled?

It takes far greater strength to go alone than rely on a boss to pay the wages and deliver the grief. – I mean, why? Why can't you live the dream, why can't you get paid for this, and why do you have to be so bloody normal?

And then there's the knowing I've made a difference in my life which means a lot.

I understand now why I'm like I am. Any different, and I'd have been caught, and in forty years time be wondering what I'd actually achieved in my working life.

Sorry, but no thanks.

We are all born with dreams; some choose to either pass them off as crazy schemes, or are forgotten in the rush to make the two point four children. Our dreams are our true path, anything else is just a diversion.

And when it comes to thinking I'm shy, ugly, messed up. I'm not messed up, I've had problems for sure, but that's not a warrant for such harsh words. I'm me, Richard.

People imposed their thoughts upon me. I took them in and my belief system altered dramatically, but now I'm changing, I'm throwing out what was said because I don't want it anymore. Whoever planted the thoughts can have them back, I'm now working from my original belief, the one I was born with.

So time for change. Goodbye to the shy Richard and hello to the confident one.

I'm not a bad person, I'm no freak either. Okay, I'm different from others, but thank God I am, who would want to be like Mr Joe Average anyhow?

I'll strive for my dream and become published. I was told I had one in a million chance of success, well that's fine, because that's all I need. One chance. One single chance.

A bit of a difference. And it's rather like receiving praise from someone you trust. Like I said before, that nice warm feeling in the pit of your stomach. - Do this enough times, and your belief system changes and the world seems brighter. It might have been a sunny day outside before, but because you had such a heavy cloud up there, you failed to notice this. Things are starting to look different already.

Exercise: - *'Now it's your turn. Glance over the negative and put everything in the positive. After, I want you to read the positive everyday for the next week. Don't doubt it, just believe it.'*

A week on

It can be quite traumatic, rewriting negative to positive and re-reading the real you in a positive, but you'll soon see how rewarding this can be, and the boost it will give your overall confidence level.

Now I want to take you on a stage further, to look back. By looking back we can deal with the 'Big Problems'. But I only want you to go back two months to start with. This should get you in the groove and ultimately ready for the 'Big one', but that's running, and we're walking for now. So, if you're ready.

Exercise: <u>A</u> – *'Write down everything that has grieved you in the past couple of months, along with all the destructive thoughts you have had about yourself.'*

Exercise: <u>B</u> – *'Like before, turn this round to the positive and read over the next week.'*

The next step

Because I can't gauge exactly where you are after the past exercises, it's difficult for me to judge when you should move to *'The 'Big' One.'* So my advice is, sense how you feel. If you don't feel strong enough as yet, don't worry, go back over the previous exercises until you do, otherwise move on.

'Our Emotion Engine' chapter will also be of use here. Not forgetting **Bach flower remedies, talking with a trusted friend, and positive self talk.**

Summary

Tick

Box

☐Small step **BIG STEP.** This is a new way of thinking, it can take time to adjust.

☐Carry out the here and now exercise to help remove your destructive thoughts.

☐Put back in the positive and keep re-reading for at least a week.

☐Now do the same but with the past couple of months exercise.

☐Don't lose heart, if it doesn't come easy, take your time. This is not a test.

☐Everyday is a new day, and it's never too late to start again.

☐Move on to the next chapter only when you feel it's the right time for you.

☐Remember, 'YOU ARE SAFE.'

- 21 -

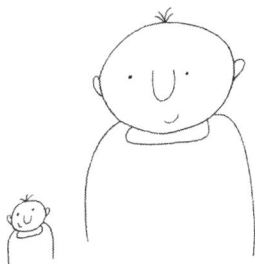

THE 'BIG' ONE

This is it, I want the full story. I've witnessed you coming a long way since the outset of this book, and now you're feeling stronger, it's time to deal with your past.

So please, take your pen in hand and don't hold back, I want everything from up there in that head of yours. Start from very first memory and take it all the way to present day. You might want to make notes first, that's fine, but I personally found it easier to just start and see what came out. Whichever way you choose, relax and just let it flow.

And one other point. It doesn't have to be Shakespeare. And you don't have to show anyone else if you don't want to. People can be very destructive, especially family when they read reality like this. Normally because they are deeply involved, and they can't face up to how they made you feel. Which means it's a good idea to keep your writing out of sight, that's unless you have a true friend who understands you, otherwise lock it safely away.

Remember, this is you. The real you on paper. How you hear, feel, see, taste, and smell, our five senses. Recall every one of them if you can, and try and paint a vibrant picture in words, because the more detail you can muster, the more ultimate power it shall have for you.

Note. – *'When writing, it doesn't have to be perfect or come in any particular order. So don't worry about the quality of the writing, only about getting the contents on paper.'*

🕯Flower remedies to take: Honeysuckle, Walnut, Elm, Gentian, Larch, and Wild Oat.

Some Pointers:

○Whatever comes into your head write it down.

○Don't edit. Keep writing. The pen must be moving at all times.

○Start from the very beginning even if you think it has no relevance.

○Try and use every sense. A smell, a feeling. Include everything and make it come alive.

○The power is in the detail.

○Don't criticise yourself. What's come out on paper is the right content for this moment in time.

○There is no wrong or right way to do this exercise.

○Don't be afraid to feel emotions when writing this. If you cry, become angry, disappointed, let it come out. This is part of the healing process.

○Don't show anyone else. You could be opening yourself up further for damaging comments if you do.

〇When you can't think of anything else, pen down and congratulate yourself on a job well done.

So now's come the time to pick up your writing instrument and begin, and as you write, you'll find your mind will release more and more, making this easier for you. But don't be surprised if the emotions come. I cried a lot during my story, things came back like it were yesterday, my written story became my reality once again and the flood gates opened. But why?

The answer, I hadn't really cried in the past. Sure there were moments, but I used to talk the problems over and over in my mind, which locked them tight inside, I needed to let them go. Which is something you've learnt by now. If something bothers you, don't let it fester within, either sort it out in a sensible way, by talking to somebody, or release the anger in a safe controlled manner, e.g. punch a pillow or write a letter. Because releasing emotions is very healing.

So here is your big chance. A new start. Keep with the flower remedies and positive self talk, work your way steadily through, and in the long term you are going to feel the difference.

The Task. – *'Now write your own story. Start with first memories and take it all the way to present time. Good luck.'*

Summary

Tick

Box

☐Offloading our negative past unlocks the future.

☐Use the most comfortable method to write your story.

☐Put as much detail in as you possibly can.

☐Clearing past negatives from your head, leaves space for positive thoughts and opportunities. – Eases anxiety.

☐This is very powerful; remember to keep taking your remedies.

☐You may feel tired and under the weather after completing this task, but don't give up, this will get you better.

☐Take time out after, and remember, be easy on yourself.

☐Congratulate yourself on a task well done.

☐'YOU ARE SAFE.'

- 22 -

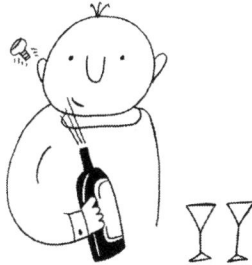

A Triumph!

Good work. Reward yourself for achieving this amazing feat. Don't worry about reading it over and understanding what you have written just yet, that will come in a moment, just lay back and relax. Bask in your total success.

Think champagne corks popping, hear people around you cheering and showering you with all the objects you have ever wanted. Punch the air in jubilation and shout this:

'YES, I'VE DONE IT, NOBODY CAN STOP ME NOW! GOODBYE PANIC, HELLO NEW ME.'

This is an important part of the process. For some time now you have been busily working away in your chosen place, bringing back all the crud that has made you as ill as you are today. You're probably feeling overwhelmed with the varied emotions that came over when writing such a difficult story, but you did it. You stared your demons head long in the face and never winced or looked away. You wrote down what needed to be said, and by rewarding yourself, you'll feel better and enjoy a real sense of achievement.

By writing it down, you've just identified all the problems you have with family or friends, and there it is, right in front of you in black and white. You have a record to make changes with, and most importantly, you can come to understand the reasons for feeling so bad, and with it, remove the power of those negative thoughts that have been racing around your mind for so long. You have taken them from up there, in your head, and put them down there, on paper. That's a big step.

Now put the work somewhere safe and close this book. I want you to go for a walk. Stretch those legs and breathe in the fresh air around you. Notice your surroundings, and start to believe exactly what you have managed to do here. - And just think, what a difference it will make to your life and those around. - Smile. However much your body pains, say this to yourself over and over.

'I AM WILLING TO CHANGE.'

Now go. – Go on, I can still see you.

Analysis & reprogramming

So, I trust you had a nice walk. Feels good doesn't it. Maybe you felt some achievement while strolling along admiring the scenery. Maybe there was an overwhelming feeling mixed with uncertainty where you are going, but don't worry. However disorientated you might feel at times, however swirling the thoughts, we need to get a grip on them. We need to understand and find you, the confident you, the one who'll beat this hell and come shining through the murk ready for anything. Now, take a deep breath and let's continue.

You'll probably by now have a fair idea what's been the major contributor to your problems just by writing them down. You'll be able to identify repeated types of people you have come into contact with that have made you feel a particular way, or circumstances that have gotten so big, your body begins a panic routine seemingly without your control. Anxiety strikes, making you want to run from a troubled moment like the cave man in the fight or flight explanation, and now we begin to understand the link between the two better. Although we're not escaping from a drooling sabre tooth tiger, that is clear. We might as well be, for the deep sensations we come under when the fear trigger is switched, are just as overwhelming.

Deciding when to go back into the lion's den

And now I come against that limitation again; to guide you personally. Only you can decide when to re-enter the lion's den and face what's been troubling you for all this time. But note, this is a major clearing for you, so revisit the chapters on healing and Bach flower remedies before doing anything else. Because re-reading what you've written can be hard, and no matter how strong you think you feel, it can be surprising the effect it will have upon you.

Let me say this however. Don't be in too much of a rush to move on because you want the panic to go. Remember, it takes many things to heal yourself, and while you're working on areas other than this exercise, it's a good time to let the writing cool off. So when you do come to tackle it, the negative power it has against you will be dramatically reduced.

🦁Flower remedies to take:

Rescue Remedy and Elm.

(For terror and panic, along with feelings of being overwhelmed).

PAB – (Positive Affirmation Builder)

Now you've made the decision to go forward, let's look closer at our writing. Take a fresh piece of paper, a pen, and I want you to draw a line down the middle. Label the left column *'Inner/Outer conflict.'* Where inner conflict would be what you perceive yourself within, e.g. 'I can't cope with life.' Outer is the thoughts others subject towards you, such as a put down, e.g. 'You'll never amount to anything.'

Work through your writing and take each conflict in turn and fill in the form. You might have to have a few sheets of paper to get it all in, that doesn't matter. What does, is you getting everything down. By leaving some out, you'll run the risk of them coming back and all your hard work will become less effective. So double check, and once satisfied everything has been included, head the second column *'New thought.'*

Okay, this is where we start to bring in the new patterns that will change you forever. Its adjusted thinking, but we'll do this in two stages, and the first is simplicity in itself. For example:

Inner/Outer conflict	New thought
I hate myself.	*I don't hate myself. In fact I love myself and who I've become.*
My primary school teacher picked on me & made me feel stupid.	That was just her opinion of me, it's not my reality. I can do anything.
To give up on myself.	*That would be a waste.* *I have so much to do.*

Get the idea? Don't worry if you can't quite get the hang of it straight away, with a little practice, you'll soon grasp the idea. And anyhow, you can always go back over the first ones and rewrite them if you so wish. But by the end, sitting in front of you you'll have a precise record of your problems and all the correct re-programming specially tailored for maximum effect. Use them regularly, and then something wonderful will happen over the coming weeks.

Now before I tell you how, it might be a good idea for me to explain why the thoughts you have now control you like they do. For starters, imagine you are a small child again, imagine your mother and father are berating you for not doing your homework and send you to your bedroom without any tea. But instead, you hang around outside the door and listen to their conversation putting you down, saying you're useless and will never amount to anything, and maybe they should have another child to make up for the waste of space they have.

It's certain you're going to feel pretty cut up hearing your own parents say those sort of things about you. You're going to be angry at first, but that conversation will go round your head, time and time again reinforcing its power, and before you know it, what your parents said in the heat of the moment, has set solid, and it starts rewriting your belief system about yourself.

And whenever you do something wrong, your mind will instantly pluck these put downs from your memory and they'll replay again and again. Take this forward a few years, and how do you expect to react if someone puts you down in front of your face? Tearful? Anger? You hate yourself? Think yourself as useless? Want to run in fear of other people thinking you're thick, a waste of space, not worthy of being here?

But only if you could have seen the original remarks for what they were. Opinions and not your reality. - Over the years we take on board what people say, and this re-programmes the mind with their opinions, until we ourselves use the same condescending words towards ourselves. When this happens, we become our own worst enemy. We add to this faulty belief system and keep berating ourselves.

And self berating over a long period is highly destructive, but we can reverse this. Just think the last time you did something you were really proud of and somebody came along and said you'd done a really good job. You felt great, light on your feet, and there was a heightened level of confidence within, making you feel as though you could conquer the entire planet if you so wished.

So for the second stage, take your new beliefs from the chart and read them throughout the day, or whenever you find yourself slipping into negative thinking.

By doing this, the negative belief system will be pummelled so hard by good productive thoughts; eventually it won't take any more, and shatter into thousands of tiny pieces. When that happens, you'll sweep the negative away and put it out with the garbage.

ꝶ⌾Take flower remedies:

Chestnut Bud and Larch.

Congratulate Yourself = Lifted Mood

Summary

Tick

Box

☐Congratulate yourself. This is a major step forward.

☐Go for a walk and clear your mind.

☐Tell yourself repeatedly: 'I am willing to change.'

☐Only return to the lion's den when you feel strong enough.

☐Use **PAB** (**P**ositive **A**ffirmation **B**uilder) and break those negative thoughts. Repeat the positives over in your mind throughout the day.

☐Ignore the negatives. Scribble over them with a pen so you can't see them anymore.

☐Go back over the healing programme whenever required. It is not a sign of weakness having to cover old ground, but a good way of clearing the negative so it won't bother you again.

☐Refer to chapter, *'Overall Plan'* for guidance.

☐Remember, 'YOU ARE SAFE.'

SPIRAL OF DEPRESSION

I THINK ABOUT OPPORTUNITIES I'VE MISSED

I FEEL DOWN, DISAPPOINTED, ANGRY

I BLAME MYSELF FOR THESE PROBLEMS

I FEEL MORE DEPRESSED

I CAN'T SEE A WAY OUT

I FEEL HOPELESS

THE JOURNEY TOWARDS SUCCESS

I HAVE BEEN THROUGH THE PAST RUBBISH FOR A REASON

I'VE LEARNT THROUGH MY MISTAKES

REALISATION: THE BIG JOURNEY IS MADE WITH MANY SMALL STEPS

I CAN SEE MY DREAM AS IF IT WAS REAL

I CAN SEE WHAT I NEED TO DO TO MAKE MY DREAM A REALITY

EVERY DAY IS A DAY CLOSER TO WHAT I WANT

I CAN DO IT

I BELIEVE IN MYSELF AND EVERYTHING I DO

I TAKE POSITIVE ACTION

I BRING SUCCESS AND JOY INTO MY LIFE

- 23 -

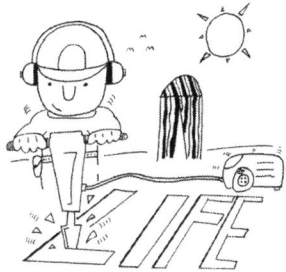

Restructuring your Life

A compilation of ways to get yourself better

Sounds scary doesn't it? But it doesn't have to be. Think it more like a fantastical new journey with endless possibilities. Recall the feeling when you left full time education and the world was out there to be conquered. You felt pretty optimistic back then didn't you. In fact, you couldn't wait to find a job and bring in a decent wage. This was a chance to do something worthwhile, fulfill all your hopes and aspirations and show who you really are.

The art of Restructuring is all about recapturing that time over again, another chance to put the record straight and start where you meant to; but for some reason didn't, or perhaps was sidetracked somewhere along the way. It's about finding that old dream again, dusting it down and going for what you want. It's about finding the inner strength. Realising this is your time, a period in your life that should be grasped with both hands and utilised for self improvement. -Yes, it might seem hard to grasp right now, especially when feeling unwell, but believe me as you get better this will all make sense. The world you thought was you will have changed. - You'll see the light. And it's going to look far brighter than you ever imagined possible.

But before you get to this crossroad, or are standing there deciding which path to take, you may feel emotional and wonder how you'll cope. It's understandable, old thought patterns can emerge, yet only if you let them will they drag you down. But with the correct handling, you can, and will, overcome. After all these are only thoughts. The Bach flower remedies will be of use here.

> ℞ Remedies to use: Elm, Larch, Gentian, Wild Oat, and Cerato.

Life's one big rush

The first thing for you is to slow everything down. The tidying up will be there tomorrow, the dirty dishes will still be there, just like the scabby bit of paintwork which you've been meaning to paint for ages, will still be there. Relax, sit back and watch trashy T.V. and DVDs, listen to music, and take long hot soaks in the bath with some aromatherapy oil. Your body needs this down time desperately, it's screaming out for rest, yet that busy racing mind of yours is only adding to the problem. And soon, BANG! – People we have an overload situation here.

Anxiety levels are high already. By dashing around, the body produces more adrenaline and the symptoms worsen. Soon enough, the pain and worry you have created upon yourself is too much, and you either have another attack, or you have to stop, unable to do anymore because you're riddled with anxiety.

By resting and controlling your breath, you can reduce symptoms, allowing the body to recognise what it feels like to be running on lower levels of anxiety. Because you've been running so high for so long, without realising it, your body thinks this state is normal. It doesn't remember the calm placid you, which is why you need to re-educate.

Day time relaxation exercise

I don't know your work circumstances, but whether you're employed, unemployed, or self employed, find the time to sit alone for five minutes. Clear your mind from the stresses of the day. Breathe, and relax. Do this at every opportunity. Tea and lunch breaks are ideal for this, yet you don't have to do this in front of your work colleagues who might laugh. Instead use a store room, or even a toilet cubicle, and no one will be the wiser. Just find the time and bring calm back into your life.

Afternoon exercise

Sit down and leave everything until tomorrow. Obviously apart from cooking, unless you can get away with that as well, do nothing. Don't think about how to get better, and try not to dwell on how you feel. Immerse yourself in a good film, eat a good meal, have a long soak in the bath, and finish off with an early night. Do this as many times a week as possible to begin with, after that, when you feel the need.

'Take one day at a time. Don't worry about what might happen tomorrow, because it might never happen.'

Both exercises might be difficult for a while, and hence, it might feel strange doing nothing at first. But fight the guilt that comes with the, 'I must do something' feeling. This time is for you, and you alone. You've been running on low batteries for too long now, so it's time for rest.

'Remember to praise yourself for taking time out. It actually takes more courage to stand up and say, 'I'm having a day off', than be pushed along by the crowd.'

Thoughts & actions. How they affect us and what to do about them

Tips:

At night, sleep without any pillows so you lay flat. This unblocks energy which otherwise would be stored in the head. Consequently reduces headaches and tension.

<u>Add Rescue Remedy and Rock Water to your bath.</u> – (For being hard on yourself). Tell tale symptoms of stress are: Stiff neck, and general tension around the shoulders and chest area.

Taking the power out from previous scenarios – When panic attacks happen, and you associate certain places or situations with having an attack. You either avoid them altogether, slowly closing in your world, or, you can stand and fight.

To beat this, you must do the latter.

For example, when I was suffering from regular attacks, I visited the Chinese medical centre in Norwich. The doctor there felt my pulse, then he looked at me and asked, 'Is there any history of heart disease in your family?'

Freaked? I was terrified. My mind raced wildly conjuring up all kinds of painful death scenarios. 'I was going to die' I told myself repeatedly, I was actually going to die. – But what evidence did I have? – In short, I panicked.

Driving home my heart was doing a fine impression of the engine's pistons running the car. I became hot and sweaty, chest pains beyond belief which only fuelled my panic further. - Now to cut a long story short, every time I merely thought about going to Norwich, the anxiety kicked in. I just had to step out the back door with the intention, and the pains would begin.

To start with, I'd shy away from this and back off, returning inside the house to recover. But I quickly realised how this was trapping me, and the only way was to force myself to face this thing head on. I had to re-introduce myself to the situation on my terms.

It hurt a great deal. But however much it hurts, however long it takes, keep going. You must do this if you're ever going to have a chance of beating this. That's why I'd suggest for the first few times take a friend along with you for moral support. It will become easier this way, because having someone with you, the chances are you are less likely to panic.

Only, don't go full out, go quarter of the way to your destination. And when this becomes tolerable, go half way, and so on. Eventually the pains and fear will diminish, and you'll find travelling doesn't bother you anymore.

'Remember to take Bach flower Rescue Remedy throughout.'

That takes care of travelling to a destination, but what about a situation you're wondering. Just get used to them in small doses. Half an hour perhaps to start with, then extending these problematic times further, proving to yourself you can do it. Remember to congratulate yourself on your achievements, however small they may be. Think, *'yeah, I did that. I am getting over this.'*

Soon you'll be able to deal with these situations, and what seemed like survival at first, will turn into enjoyment. The fears drop, by replacing them with the knowledge you can handle the situation in your stride. The panic entered through the same door, now you can shut it out, rewriting the brain's hard drive with positive. - *See 'To Walk the Devil's Yard.'*

Late nights – Simply, these should be avoided for now. Tiredness makes matters worse. You only have to think back to how jittery and anxious you become when you're tired. How everything hurts more, how situations and people are more difficult or impossible to deal with, and this makes sense. Concentration also wanes, which is why sleep deprivation is serious. So take note. We charge best at night. The hours before twelve are our most beneficial, before tailing off in the small hours. So try to get some sleep starting around half nine – ten o'clock. And don't think one night will be enough. It's accumulative. Which means you are going to have to keep it up for a while. After that, you'll be the judge on how much you need.

Ways for ensuring a good night's sleep:

O Write down all your problematic thoughts. This clears the mind and brings calmness.

O Meditate half an hour before bedtime.

O Take a Bach flower remedy. Your practitioner will be of help here.

O Have a hot bath, pamper yourself. Light some incense sticks in your bedroom.

○ Listen to some nice music.

○ Have a partner give you a massage with some aromatherapy oils.

Pacing yourself - This can be difficult. Easier if you're self employed or retired, because you can control your day's work load. Otherwise fast frantic work raises stress, which is obviously to be avoided. Signs you're overdoing it can come with headaches, chest pains, a feeling of high agitation and sickness. A sudden moment of deep fear that the worst is going to happen is normal. But with a steady breathing technique, anxious feelings are overcome, yet will return all too quickly if calm is not maintained.

Employed people however, need to discuss this with the boss. I realise you won't want to be singled out with special needs; there's nothing worse than feeling an outsider from your work colleagues when you're feeling vulnerable already. But believe me, by discussing the problem and making someone understand, it can release enormous pressure. However, if you're unlucky to have a boss who is more worried about profit margins than his staff, I know what I'd do. Walk. Whatever you stand to lose, nothing is worth damaging your health over, and you must remember that.

Circumstances might have to change, but what would you rather have? A flash car, a nice big house? Or good health? And anyway, what use are they if you're not well enough to enjoy them. These things can always be bought again. You can't.

Overly berating yourself – The anger can come from deep down and be immensely strong. So strong in fact, you wouldn't stand for it if someone treated you in such a way. So why do you inflict such anger upon yourself?

What you're actually doing is taking on the role of all the people who said nasty things to you, or about you behind your back. These words have come so strong, strengthened by repetition in your own mind, you've now taken on the role of thinking them as true. 'Maybe so and so was right. - He said I was useless,' and so on.

Whether it's someone saying it to you, or you to yourself, the effect has become the same, emotions come with physical sickness.

Think of it as though you're telling off a small child. That child is vulnerable, it feels pain easily when you're horrible, and by doing this over and over, how do you think this child is going to feel? How will he view the outside world if he feels like a reject, a misfit, someone who's really a waste of space and has no hope of making anything of his life? You think he will be strong, well adjusted after years of battering like that? - It's now time to nurture that small child within you. *'Be kinder to __YOU__. Build yourself up.'*

Worrying too much before the event – We all do it, what if so and so is there, I don't know if I can cope. What if the plane is late? What if I have an attack on the plane? What if the plane is delayed? What if….?

In anxiety driven mode this can become so terrifying we back out and stay safe. We cancel appointments and retreat, telling ourselves all sorts of nasty putdowns, because we can't cope with something simple like getting on a train. But we needn't, you can cope in the right mind set.

I mentioned in a previous chapter about visualisation. Our minds cannot determine between imagination and real life. For example, ever had one of those dreams that have put you in a good or bad mood, even though it wasn't real? Or one that really made you think. Or one where you lost someone and you felt grief for that imaginary person? - That's the mind being unable to recognise imagination.

So here's what we do. Carry out this type of exercise once a day, or if you're doing something at short notice, repeatedly before departure.

Example scenario

You have to get on a plane; let's say Geneva for a business meeting. You're flying business class as per normal, and you have with you an overnight bag. You'll be picked up from home by taxi, which will deliver you and your luggage outside the airport ready to check in.

Visualisation exercise

I want you to start from the moment you wake up. Imagine you're going through to the bathroom to wash, toilet, and clean your teeth etc. Now imagine getting dressed, having breakfast, and readying yourself for the taxi. See that taxi arrive, pick up your bag and walk out. Not forgetting to lock the door behind you.

You say to yourself, 'I am in total control.'

In the taxi you relax in the knowledge you are making good time and there is no need to hurry. Imagine the driver pulling up outside the airport. Exit the taxi, pay the driver before heading for the check in counter. Check in, smile at the girl behind the counter, and thank her kindly (we still keep manners even in imaginary land).

It's about time for a drink and maybe a bite to eat. Stop over at one of the restaurants and pick something out, whatever takes your fancy.

But don't forget to ask the woman behind the counter for a drink, remembering you must stay away from caffeine.

You pay and calmly take a seat, after which you notice there's a rack with some newspapers on. You lean over and pick one, relaxing, you have plenty of time.

You say to yourself, 'I am safe and relaxed, there is nothing to fear.'

Later you stand up, notice it's time to move through passport control and into the departure lounge.

You hand your passport over, and the man raises an eyebrow at the picture you wish you'd never have used, yet was still better than the other four. He hands you a boarding ticket and you continue. Security checks your hand luggage and you are scanned by a machine; but of course all is in order.

You take a seat in the departure lounge, deciding not to bother looking around the shops. Instead you watch the people milling about from the seat you have chosen.

You see a woman wearing a red dress, she looks glamorous,and you swear she's a model or a famous actress. Then a man in a suit sits beside you and asks for the time, which you give willingly. The man thanks you kindly and comments on the good weather before reading a rather crumpled yesterday's paper.

You take little notice, but still can't help wondering why anyone would want to look back over old news.

You say to yourself, 'from today I only look forwards.'

You're called. You stand and gather your things up before queuing. The queue is very long, but the wait doesn't cause any bother because they are not going to leave without you. You have plenty of time.

You say to yourself, 'I have no reason to panic. I am in control of my life.'

Eventually you hand over the boarding pass; you travel down a long tunnel which bears left at the bottom. A couple of stewards are standing in the planes hatch busily welcoming people aboard.

You glance at the ticket, just to double check the seat number you'll occupy for the flight. One of the stewards kindly directs you, and within a minute you're buckling in.

You say to yourself, 'I am safe.'

The seat next door is already occupied by a woman who says hello warmly, naturally you return the greeting, and then engage in a conversation about the lovely red dress she is wearing.

I could have added more detail and continued until the journey's end, but you can do that for yourself. The point being, whatever the trip, venue, or meeting, you can run through the whole event in your mind, making sure when it actually comes to the real thing, it will be water off a duck's back. Your mind will have become used to the trip, so consequently nothing shall worry it.

Recognising the signs you're over doing it - To keep this simple, when your body hurts, don't go pushing it. You've pushed it so hard in the past it needs a rest. Pain, where panic attacks are concerned, is an indicator to take time out. You'll come to recognise the early warning signs, which will become an invaluable tool for coping and healing yourself.

But I'm not good enough thinking – For me, on a scale of 1-10, I'd say this was an eleven. People tell you different. They say how good you are, but because of the past negative thoughts you've been having, their comments literally bounce off that wall you have built for yourself. You desperately want to believe them, but inside you feel different. You look upon whatever you say and do as being useless, and when you do something of worth, what do you say?

I'll do better next time. Nothing you do satisfies your mind. You can't believe why people like you because you class yourself as a freak, a no hoper, who might as well reside to the fact nothing will become of you.

But you are good enough. If it's proof you require, just think of someone you helped today, or yesterday, or last week. You reached out to them in an hour of need. When they wanted somebody to help, you stepped forward and lent a hand. Nobody waved a fist of readies in your face. You helped because you wanted to. You knelt down and picked up that old lady's groceries, which she'd accidentally spilled over the floor, because you care. And people who care, those who take the time out from personal gain to help a fellow human, are higher than mere just good enough. That's approaching God like material.

But you feel you have achieved nothing in your life. I understand this. So now's the time to prove yourself. Either you sit worrying about wasting time, and getting nowhere fast, or you make a stand. You bid for the very thing that will prove you are worthy of the title you think you're not. – And for the record, just beating this panic alone will be an amazing achievement in itself.

My big achievement was writing this book. Yours might be something similar. I don't know. Maybe you've always wanted to help people, but this type of negative thought pattern prevented you in the past.

Yet, if you're really truly want to do something, if it's what your heart truly desires. Then go for it. Break free, prove you can do it. The strength is there, trust your inner dream will provide. Because if it wasn't there, you'd have no dream. And if you had no dream, the burning urge to do something would be vacant. And whilst this is not the case, I guess you better go and do something about it.

Say regularly: *'I approve of myself and everything I do.'*

Slaying the dragon within – My nan said this to me once. It was something my dad's brother said many times before his untimely death, which made me believe he too was suffering from what I found deep in myself. The Dragon being the fear that had to be slayed every time he wanted to do something, otherwise he felt too disempowered, unable to face whatever was waiting outside.

267

It can help to visualise your dragon inside. If you don't want to slay him, (he might have a nice face), just coax him into a large cage with a piece of juicy red meat, then lock the door behind him. Once done, do what you have to do without the negative thinking.

Negative thinking will only start the worst scenarios spinning, the dragon will bust out, and before you know it hot grill your behind.

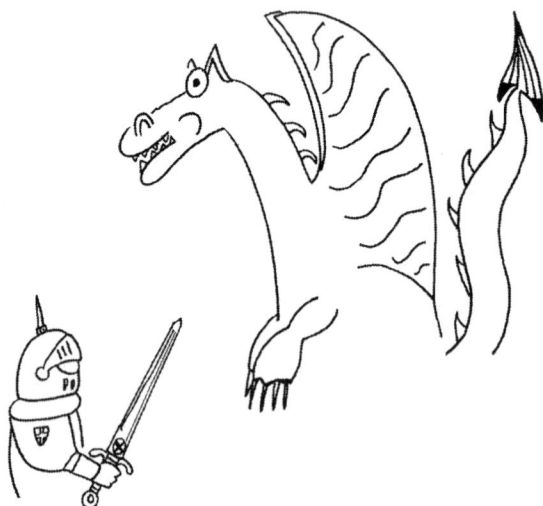

Negative thinking = Negative results

Positive thinking = Positive results

Forgetting the past - The negative past has a powerful grasp upon us. We know this, because whenever we're all alone and nothing occupies us, we turn to what has fallen before. We dredge the past back, we begin to dissect it, why this happened, why so and so said that, even though he knew it would be hurtful, and so on. Like a bower-constrictor, it squeezes our very being. We become depressed, pained, short of breath, and tearful. Our minds race unable to understand. - But really, should we bother doing this time and time again?

No - I mean, what's the point? The past has gone, along with all those comments or actions people said or did. Do you think they are thinking about how they treated you? Dwelling over the past in deep misery because of what they have done?

Of course they don't. They can't remember. Which comes full circle again to berating yourself. Although unintentional; by bringing these thoughts and emotions back, you are in fact creating what can only be called mental torture upon yourself. Release that grip of the past, and look forward to the future. In the future, anything can happen. And the past? Time to let it go.

Like an old banger of a car, discard and buy a new one. Forget the old faithful which transported you to and from work, and look forward to driving the new sparkly machine outside. You are the sparkly machine revving to go, floor the throttle and take it to the stars.

Say: *'I happily release the past knowing it has no power over me anymore.'*

And: *'As I look forward to the future, I smile towards my new beginnings.'*

'Decide to remember the good times, but banish the bad ones forever.'

Harnessing the dream and how it can adversely affect those around you

This is something you might be up against. I'm not saying this is the case, because there are those of you who will have the love and support to grow how you so wish. But I'm going to stick my neck out here and say more will be on the negative side. I say that, because normally the route of the problem comes from those closest around you. The ones who hit the heart the most, and for the longest. That's where the pain often originates, leaving you no choice but to stand and battle with what's been imposed upon you.

You want to stand up and do something different, but some people will insist on being less than encouraging of your idea, by giving you all the reasons why it can't possibly work.

For you, it's a test of willpower. Are you going to listen to these people, or are you going to ignore them, and continue with what you know in your heart is right?

You must stick to your inner feelings, otherwise you'll be working from somebody else's belief system, and when that happens, conflicts rise within you and creates anger. Especially if things don't turn out as well as they should.

> ✌🔘Remedies to take are: Century, Larch, Elm, Gentian, and Cerato.

But not all people are necessarily bad, they might be overprotective of you, and don't want to see you putting yourself at risk with such an idea. They genuinely care and would rather see you do something where the outcome is guaranteed. Which is understandable. You've worked your way through very anxious times lately, and they just don't want to see you go down that hole again. – But you have to think, was it the nice safe route that contributed to your problems in the first place? And then, would doing something you've always wanted create the excitement within, and make the outside world look a better place than it currently does?

If the answer is yes to both, then you know what to do. Overprotection doesn't help anybody. Life is full of risk taking, and how do you know if something will work or not if you haven't tried it in the first place?

Then there will be those who will feel threatened by your new found strength and power.

Some feel in control when you're all wobbly and need their assistance in everything you do. They are your crutch in life, and as long as this continues, they are happy. They have the reigns and they can control their environment and feel masterful.

But remember, the person in control is often weaker than the person who is gaining in strength. As you become the person you were born to be, they see you as a threat towards their reign, and may use all their power to bring you down to a level they can handle.

Quite often it's not because they don't want you to get on, but because they are trying to protect you in their own way. They strongly believe their opinion is the right one, and whatever you say is going to be dismissed. Unless you are in agreement of course. - But take heart, the more you persist in your new way of thinking, they will stop trying to influence you, allowing you more space with what you are trying to achieve.

'To bring greater strength along with a willingness to stand your ground, use the remedy Centuary.'

Say: *'I am striving to be the best I can be. My Dream can be my reality.'*

Envisage your 'BIG DREAM' by getting hold of a regular note book and start writing it down. Always carry it with you, so when inspiration does strike, the moment will never be lost. Write as though today you are going into action. Rather like a major battle plan. Make every detail count. Work constantly here, and your dream shall clarify to the point you can almost touch it. Thus empowering you with the kind of confidence to finally go for what you desire. (And remember, the 'BIG DREAM' is about the whole picture, not just a small part like making money).

Don't ever be bullied into something you don't want to do, or be a slave for others around you - One of the feelings imposed upon ourselves is guilt. Guilt is used to great effect by others to get what they want out of you. We've all heard sayings like, 'come round for Christmas, it might be granny's last.' The same line that's been trooped out for the past umpteen years and you've come to expect the old girl's dead and buried, until the following Christmas reminds you otherwise.

This might be a rather tame example, but guilt can be used to make us feel bad about ourselves. That we're weak, shy, and unsociable. Especially if we don't attend a particular function. The truth is, we're weak if we don't stand up and say, 'no, I don't want to go.' It's all about doing what you want to do, and not doing what everybody expects of you.

Another example. You sit there at a party wanting to be somewhere else. The only reason you went was because a partner or family member said you had to go. For Doris's sake. Making out you'd be the only person she could talk to. Except old Doris is having a whale of a time with skinny Bob from down the road, and quite frankly, couldn't care less if you were there or not. You want to leave, but instead you end up clock watching until it's time to go.

Sound familiar? – Don't worry, as you increase in strength, you'll be able to say that magic word, *'No'* and mean it. You'll begin to ditch any feelings of guilt when they try and impose the same old tired guilt trips, and by doing this, you'll feel like the boss and not the slave.

Which makes it a good time to mention boundaries. Our boundaries are often within the home and involve those closest to us. So, try delegating some of your chores. Just because you have done them in the past, doesn't mean you always have to do them in the future. Learn to say *'No'* and not feel guilty. What you are starting to do here is honour yourself and your time.

By doing this, it is a very empowering act, and you'll soon start to feel more confident and assertive in yourself.

Only, don't be surprised if there are a few challenges at first. Little Jimmy may get angry if he has to tidy his room and help wash up after dinner. But the good news is, he will start to recognise and honour your boundaries if you stay strong and don't back down. Any chink of weakness and he'll play on that and try and wear you down. – *'So, stay strong, don't feel guilty, and it's perfectly okay to say 'No.'*

The same goes for holding boundaries at work. If you've always done everything, colleagues will expect this of you, and won't even think about doing one of your jobs. You have to make your boundaries clear and enforce them, otherwise people will take advantage.

Remember:

'Conforming to others against our wishes brings us down. Standing our ground brings great strength.'

Why can't you be like ordinary people? - Do we have to? I mean, really. Do we? Is there some sacred book which says we have to live the same as everybody else?

We can live how we want. And as long as we keep within the law, there is nothing saying when you leave school you must find a job in the rat race, get married, buy a nice house, fill it with a couple of kids and purchase a people carrier to move them about in. Which incidentally, you'll spend every Sunday cleaning, and then moan you don't have the time for anything else anymore.

And when you've done all that, you have to expect no time whatsoever for yourself until retirement, when you're too tired to appreciate anything. Your nine to five office job may give you no sense of achievement, and by the end, you'll sit your last days on this planet wondering what you've done of worth.

There is no book as such that says this of course. But for some reason, it has become an unwritten law that if you don't do these things, you're odd, a freak, a strange anomaly who probably needs psychiatric help.

'It takes more courage to go against the grain than it does to go with it.'

'On this earth we all have the right to do whatever we want as long as it is within the law!'

The over importance on what we own - When I was suffering, I used to think I needed a classic car so people would stop and talk to me. I made it my mission to restore these cars because it made me feel good momentarily, which meant I could face the world. Though it didn't last long. I'd look for another project. I wanted approval, but inside I became angry at myself for not doing a good enough job. That anger built until it became deep and fierce, so much so, I recognised it wasn't doing me any good. But still, there was no way of controlling it when it happened.

Healing took away this deep seated anger, along with the need for a flash looking car. I discovered people talk to me because they want to, not because the type of vehicle I drive. In truth, the majority don't care. Yes they might admire, but a minute later the moments gone, and I came to realise it's really me that matters, not a piece of motorised metal. And when that finally struck home, I also realised health is the greatest gift of all. Sure money helps, only a fool would say it doesn't. But it isn't everything. People strive solely for years to make their millions, and when it happens, they feel empty. To fill their emptiness they buy cars, yachts, villa's abroad. Do they feel satisfied? The answer, probably not. Money alone can't do that, and can never.

How many times have you walked into a shop, bought something you really wanted for ages, got the short fix, but after a while lost interest? We all do it. But now think back to when you really helped somebody, and it doesn't have to be monetary. Maybe you helped them with their garden, fixed their car, or gave a kind word. You felt good inside. And whenever you think or see that person now, it brings back that feeling. Now can a material item do that in the long term?

But money is not all bad. When shared, instead of spending on the self, that's when it makes a difference. But for some reason many make their fortune and just concentrate on where the next big deal is coming from. If only they used this money to good purpose, such as helping communities, or research and environmental issues. They'd feel great for lending a hand. Not to mention making a real difference to people's lives the whole world over.

So why in today's society have we become so enclosed within our own space? You see people readily in the supermarket who blank the cashier, and then those who stare straight through you when you give a smile, or a kind nod. Funnily, it takes a lot less energy to be calm and at peace with the world than angry. People don't respond well to anger. And anyway, those angry people are causing more harm to themselves than they actually realise. As you know from reading this book, negativity pushes others away and eats you inside.

But don't go thinking because they are like that, why should you bother to smile and say hello. Because somewhere along the line, you'll make somebody's day when otherwise they were having a bad one.

Summary

Tick

Box

◻Restructuring your life needn't be feared. It's a time for positive change.

◻Slow down and relax. Pace yourself. Recognise when you're starting to overdo things and stop for a rest.

☐Time to stop berating yourself, there's no need to be a taskmaster anymore.

☐Try not to over-worry before an event, what will be, will be.

☐Run the event over in your head beforehand to diminish the power it holds.

☐You are a good person, nobody has the right to say different.

☐As you gain strength, those around might see you as a threat. Ignore them, they have no power over you.

☐Learn to say *'NO'* - you don't have to be like everybody else.

☐Remember, it takes more courage to go up stream than be washed down.

☐Smile, be happy. Change is coming.

☐Remember, 'YOU ARE SAFE.'

- 24 -

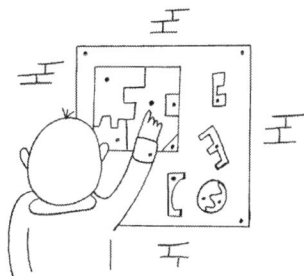

Putting the Pieces Back Together

Now I can sit back and look at what's gone before me, I think it's only right to try and clarify my story, so you the reader can see how the healing programme works. The whole process can take time, I've made this clear elsewhere, but with persistence, along with a strong determination to turn this around, comes the rewards you have been searching for for so long. I'm not trying to make this glossy, because it's not, you are dealing with real emotions here. At times they can hurt a great deal, so much so it feels like nothing on this earth. But in the positive, they can be the most uplifting part of our lives, which is why it's so important to understand them better.

For now, your emotions can seem out of control. You may be wondering how you'll ever get a true grasp. But try and not be too despondent here, stay positive, because as whirly as they may seem right now, with practice, they shall become easier and the bad times will be outweighed by the good.

'These are exciting times; you can, and will, achieve anything your heart's desire.'

A reflection on things that have passed by

Recently things turned into something I'd been dreading for a long time now. The death of my stepmother. Margaret's cancer took over her body, and there was nothing she or the doctors could do about it. I guess you could say it was her time, but that doesn't make it any easier, especially where my father is concerned.

Death is never welcome, but in this case to a degree it was. Margaret's pain had gotten so bad at times all she could do was cry, her bones where crumbling and her life diminishing. So when death did finally come knocking, there was a certain amount of release there, and I could see that clearly written across her face after she'd passed on. But for me personally, it seemed more complicated than that. As I begin to go deeper, the emotions in me are very mixed and confusing. So let me get a handle on this and try and explain.

As hard as I try, I can't get away from the simple fact I was angry about the whole deceiving thing. My father had left my mother for another woman, that I could get my head around to some degree, but he had been seeing this woman for most of my childhood years.

Yet, how could they keep a lie about their relationship and think we would just accept what they'd done? Did they just expect we'd all get on like happy families? – It seems confusing. My father made us feel bad if we didn't treat Margaret the way he thought we should, the same for her son Alex. But there was no reason we should have all been best friends, especially when we were never given the chance to say what we wanted, instead we were just told.

It was a difficult situation, that's fair to mention. But say I was given another chance. Say, by some miracle the clocks went back ten years and I was faced with the same encounter. - What would I do?

For starters, I would have been more honest. If I'd just said how I felt in the first place, instead of being nice, and skating around the problem, perhaps we would have become closer later down the line.

There has to be something said for honesty, but it's not always that easy. In fact, it's actually harder to stand up for what you believe. It's easier to get washed down the river and not rock the boat, even though the outcome is not what we actually desire.

Yes it might upset a few people to begin with, it might get their backs up so much the relationship breaks down, but think about what you are achieving here. Think about the overall picture and not the immediate reality.

So bringing it back, I can understand why my father and Margaret did what they did. Here were two people who risked everything so they could be together, who wanted to enjoy life for however long they had, and just be themselves.

I'm not saying what they did was some sordid horrid affair, just like I'm not saying I suffered panic attacks because of what they did, because that's untrue, the simple fact is, I was, and still am to some degree angry for the way we kids were treated. But I must emphasise this, the panic attacks were not caused by this fact alone, there were many other issues that needed to be dealt with to overcome the onslaught of varied emotions that ravaged inside of me.

Is this confusing? – Are you thinking you won't be able to find the answers to why your own panic attacks have struck? Does it feel as though it's one big mass of a problem and there is no way you can dissect it in this way? Or know where to even start?

Relax. The story you wrote about yourself was for a further purpose. It's also a tool for dissecting and understanding how you came to this point in your life. Yes it was angry, of course it was, there was a lot of emotional release there. But now try and step back from this in exactly the same way you did with the positive affirmation builder. Realise all this was in the past, and it holds no power over you anymore.

But firstly, let me make this clearer for you.

So here comes the big question:

Why did I have panic attacks?

Firstly let me break down the way I looked at things.

OI hated the way my parents treated me at times, all the put downs destroying my confidence.

OI hated their fighting, destabilising us as a family unit.

OI hated the fact my father had cheated on my mother and we'd all been living a delusion for a large chunk of my life.

OI hated the fact my mother makes me look about five years old in front of other people, doing her best to embarrass me or make me look stupid.

OI hated being told off for wetting the bed, being turned away in the mid of night with a strong feeling I was the cause of their anger.

○I hated school and facing people when dealing with my IBS.

○I hated how my mother got angry if I said I couldn't eat something because it upset my stomach.

○I hated feeling inferior to others because my parents made me feel this way. Telling everybody I was shy.

○I hated the way other children said I was thick.

○I hated the way my body reacted to just being alive. I felt overly anxious and that I couldn't cope with life.

○I hated meeting Margaret for the first time and my father just presuming we all should just get along.

○I hated the fact my father just disappeared with his new woman and he hardly ever made contact.

○I hated the fact it was always down to me to pop in and see my father.

○After we met Margaret, the going out for dinner trips just stopped. I felt cut off and more detached than ever.

○I hated the fact my father felt like somebody you just bumped into the street occasionally.

○I hated the fact my family never believed I could make it as a writer.

○I hated the fact all my past attempts at becoming somebody were seen as big failures. A waste of money, a waste of time. I hadn't the expertise or knowledge, they said.

○I hated being told I wasn't normal because I didn't do

what normal kids do.

○I hated being told *'I was a dirty muckworm,' or asked, 'Who would fancy that?'*

○I hated being told to get a normal job. A normal life.

○I hated feeling an outcast because I suffered from panic attacks.

○I hated the way people treated me when they found out I had difficulties.

○I hated the world along with the people who filled it, because it felt as though everybody treated me bad.

And there we have the majority of my thinking. The type of things that brought me down to a place I found it difficult to climb out of. But all that hate and anger didn't vent out. I didn't go round screaming and shouting because that's not how I am, instead it went internal. It grew inside to a point my body couldn't handle it anymore. Like a volcano I erupted, namely panic attacks.

The anger towards myself had come from the anger, dislike, and put downs others had directed at me. I hated me. The very person I should be kindest to. Yet I was the cruellest. I told myself horrid things and the continual barrage from others only compacted my faulty belief system that bit further.

But why didn't I just walk out of the situation? Why didn't I say enough's enough and get the hell out? – Because no matter how bad I felt, how bad the things people said to me, this was my comfort zone. You have to remember, the outside world was one heck of a scary place for me to venture out into, given the chance, I didn't want to be born, let alone have to deal with life. I just couldn't cope, I just couldn't understand who, or what I was meant to be.

So what was the cause of my panic? A mixture of anger and self hatred. A feeling of going nowhere and never being the person everybody else seemed to be.

I guess what I thought was *'NORMAL.'* I saw myself as not being able to cope with the type of things normal people do. Like falling into a relationship, talking to people without wanting to shy away, buying something from a shop without going beetroot red, living like others and feeling comfortable in my own skin.

It's fair to say, I hated being me. Everyone seemed okay, but me, forget it. I felt the outcast, the loser, the waste of space that shouldn't actually be here breathing valuable air. – Sounds horrid, but it was a difficult place living as Richard Hathaway. I was embarrassed being me, and because of this, it was difficult coping.

The answer? From day one honour yourself. You have not been put on this planet to serve everybody's needs twenty-four seven. You need down time, you deserve to enjoy life and feel all the pleasures that come with it. – Be kinder, stop any self berating. Understand those around better, and look to the future instead of all the past garbage, otherwise known as yesterday's news. Yes, people might have been horrid in the past, and perhaps they still are in the present. But it's your life. You can be who you want to be, no matter what anybody else says.

So when looking back at your own panic attacks after the main healing programme, take a moment to work through and come to understand why. You'll find the big picture will be easier to tackle than you might think, because everything will become clearer and the problems will ultimately lose their power.

Exercise – understanding why

Now I want you to sit down with a clean sheet of paper and do what I have just done. Write down all the problems you have come up against (refer back to your own story for this, and any pieces you wrote from the other chapters) and you'll begin to see a picture emerge and the clues to why panic became such a problem for you. – And don't worry if it doesn't smack you round the face like a wet kipper to begin with, it can take time to recognise how each piece of the jigsaw fits. But with a little working back, it will become clear.

Using myself as an example again, I could see that anger was playing a big part, so by reducing or eradicating anger from my life, the panic also diminished. I say diminished, because that was not the only problem. I needed to honour myself more and take time out without feeling guilty. I guess, look after me without trying to please everyone else all of the time.

These can be hard lessons to learn. The body feels rushed, and it can take a while to re-programme the mind so things become calmer. But without identifying where your problems come from in the first place, you are rather shooting in the dark.

Some pointers for overcoming panic attacks:

O **Honour yourself. Don't let others rule your life. And it's okay to say '_NO!_'**

O **Be kinder to yourself in everything you do. Don't beat yourself up.**

O **Change negative into positive. Say, '_I can do this,_' not, '_I can't._'**

○ Recognise your strengths and utilise them fully.

○ Recognise you are an okay person.

○ Think future not past. What's gone before doesn't have to influence you now.

○ Recognise how far you've come.

○ Recognise where your problems come from and make changes.

○ If you are angry about a person, it's okay to confront them and tell them how you feel. If this feels too much, write your feelings down for now and approach the person when you feel stronger.

○ Remember it's okay to get angry, just don't allow that anger to eat away at you.

○ And finally, relax and chill out as often as you can. A busy mind creates panic, a relaxed one gets more done and feels happy.

Reflecting back

It's not always easy to look back and see how far you've come. And I'm certainly no different. But while I write this, I can't help but feel a little pleased with myself. I've come from the pits of desperation, a place so horrid it turned my world into a living nightmare, yet I fought hard. I didn't give up because somewhere deep in my heart I knew there must be an answer.

Many a time I've sat on the edge of my bed waiting to die, the pains were telling me this, although in reality, it was me misreading what was actually happening, and blowing everything out of proportion.

Yet it's understandable. The pains were so uncomfortable, so bad, I thought about killing myself just so I could escape from what felt like torture. It felt like I couldn't escape, trapped in a dysfunctional body hemming me in with every passing hour. Words cannot describe the agony, not fully, but it was the most difficult time of my life. - Saying that, now I have come to accept what happened, put it in perspective, and I know forwards is better than backwards.

But also, by making the decision to change, and never giving up on myself, beat this. Without the desire to overcome, I'd still be stuck and wondering what life had in store for me.

And now, where has all this taken me? Into a world I thought was never possible. But here I am with a book, a light for others to follow so they too can feel what I feel, a world without panic.

Just to live without the sickness and fears is something very special. To wake up knowing I am not going to have an attack, and that my life is under my control now, instead of under some invisible demon that struck whenever it felt like it, is worth more than I can possibly say.

I can go places now and not have to worry. I can sit on the beach and watch the waves crashing in for as long as I like, I can finally be me.

Recently I took up Reiki and Spiritual healing, I've also been asked to do a talk, and this is from shy Richard who was too scared to do anything. Which all makes me feel I am worthy of being here, I'm not a waste of space, and I have a purpose to help others.

Over the many years panic has showed me many things, and for this reason, I don't regret going through it because the outcome is something so much better than I had before. I understand myself, I know what effects things have on me, and if need be, I can adjust accordingly so my health and happiness remains a priority. It's not about being selfish, because without being well I wouldn't be in the position to help those in need.

Which is why, I have to make sure number one is okay first, then act, because putting others first only builds anger and resentment, not to mention a feeling of losing a grip on where I want to go. But from this day forward, I will manage myself better day by day, and as long as I do this, panic will never return.

Nowadays I see possibilities instead of obstacles. I feel so excited with what the future holds, I just want to get stuck in and enjoy the ride. This is my future now, a new beginning where I can do whatever I want. I don't need anyone's permission, if I want to write a Sci-fi novel, I'll do it. If I want to be a success, I'll go ahead without taking notice of the people who say its not possible. This is my life, and I'll live it how I want.

The excitement builds inside of me. I see my books on shelves. I see myself signing copies around the globe. I see the success growing, and me, Richard, created all this. I didn't hang around and wait for it to fall in my lap, I worked hard, I dismissed the negative comments and pushed ahead anyway. I wanted this, I really wanted this, and now my dream has become a reality. It is possible, and I'm living proof.

So where do you go from here? How do you find that inner happiness that makes you all bubbly with a burning passion for life?

Always be patient with yourself, and acknowledge your own needs and desires without feeling guilty. Panic comes about because you don't honour yourself, you don't think you are worthy, and you worry what others may think. Change this, and panic will not be a problem anymore.

But more than anything, don't give up. You will come to feel that inner serenity and peace of mind, yet it may be a gradual process. And as the days, weeks, and months past, the feelings will subside and calmness will resume. This can be one of the hardest journeys you'll ever undertake, but it will also be the most rewarding. But remember, no other place will you find the big answers, they can only come from within.

So good luck, and don't be afraid to keep re-reading this book and using the exercises. You are not a failure by doing this. Certain aspects may require repeating until an eradication of the problem occurs, but it doesn't matter, try to go with it, and good health will be all yours. - This is your new start. – Take care and be well.

Richard.

'Look beyond the panic and strive for whatever you desire'

- 25 -

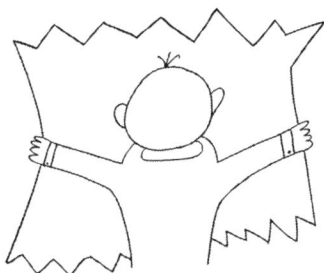

Overall Plan

When you're embarking on any journey in life, it's a nice idea to have a map of where you're going, and because of this simple fact, I've included a plan of action.

For ease, I've explained the stages in text, along with a simple to follow chart situated at the end of the chapter. Both of which correspond with the book.

Panic attack! – Something is wrong with your life. You have bought this book and this is going to be a major turning point for you. *See chapter's, 'A New Beginning', 'Introduction', and 'Survival Kit.'*

Oh my God I am going to die thinking – You are not going to die. What you're feeling are symptoms of anxiety ('The Fight or Flight response') *see chapter, 'So what is a Panic Attack?'*

Visit to the doctors – Don't worry, we all start here first. Listen to what he has to say, and when he tells you it's nothing more than anxiety, relax, because in your hands you have the perfect tool to fight it.

Recognising the symptoms for what they are – In nearly

every case, every feeling is a direct response to too much adrenaline in the body. By recognising this alone, it removes much of the power it holds over you. *See chapters, 'Sensations & Dealing with the Mental Side', and 'Coping Strategies.'*

New thinking, *'I will come to no harm'* – Reprogramming the mind from negative to positive, alters the way our body responds towards situations. Simply by saying, 'I am willing to change,' tells your brain it's time to begin work for a new you.

There are various stages of positive self talk, but in the beginning, we keep it simple, so not to overstress the body when it's in an already weakened state. *See chapter, 'A New Beginning.'*

Bach flower remedies – If there is only one thing you take away with you from reading this entire book, take the remedies. *See chapter, 'Bach Flower Remedies.'*

Control the breath - When we breathe correctly it calms the body down. When we panic, the breath comes in short rapid gasps, making us feel dreadful, (excessive adrenaline & oxygen). *See chapter, 'Survival Kit.'*

Look at diet – Stimulants such as tea, coffee, and alcohol, all become our enemy when dealing with anxiety. Watch your sugar intake.

Eating at the correct time is important too. You wouldn't leave home without any fuel in the car, the same applies for you. Run dry, and again adrenaline is produced to fuel us. We feel bad, get the shakes, and become light headed. - So eat at consistent times, nourish the body correctly, and remember to drink plenty of water. *See chapter, 'Diet and the Importance.'*

Relaxation technique - Stressed out? It only makes sense to

relax. Relaxation reminds the body how it feels to be in a state of calm. *See chapters on, 'Visualisation and Meditation – Power of the mind', 'Restructuring your Life', & 'Survival Kit.'*

Find someone I can trust to talk to – Finding someone who you can trust to talk to is a great healer. *See chapter, 'A Fallen Star.'*

Keep a diary – The diary method is the first stage in getting whatever's been racing around your mind on paper. Effectively calming your mind. *See chapter, 'Keeping a Diary.'*

Plan a simple task – Reintroducing yourself to something as basic as going down the shops can feel like world war three is breaking out within you. But through this method, you can desensitise yourself in any situation so panic never bothers you again. *See chapter, 'To Walk the Devil's Yard.'*

Plan an entire day – Through careful planning, you'll see how easy it is to control the day's events, taking out the rush that previously plagued your life. *See chapter, 'What a Difference a Day Makes.'*

Writing my story – Writing about your first memory to the here and now removes the negatives, ensuring they are buried away allowing you to tackle the future. *See chapter, 'The Big One.'*

Realisation, I can do whatever I thought I couldn't do – Believe you can do anything. The only thing that stops you is you. Other people have opinions, but if you truly believe in where you're going, nothing can stand in your way.

Recognising self worth – We all deserve to be living on this planet. Be proud of who you are.

Plan the dream – We all have a dream. Whether it be to have good health, buy a house in the sun, run the next computer empire, or just be a fantastic mum and dad. The point is, dreams are there to be fulfilled. When we don't achieve them, there's a feeling of emptiness in our lives.

Taking the step, restructuring my life – Changing lifestyle and going for what you want. The future beckons. *See chapter, 'Restructuring your Life.'*

Recognising I have control in everything I do – In the beginning our emotions feel totally uncontrollable. With a new understanding, the uncontrollable becomes controlled. **See** *chapter, 'Putting the Pieces Back Together.'*

The Path to Beating Panic and Realising your Dreams

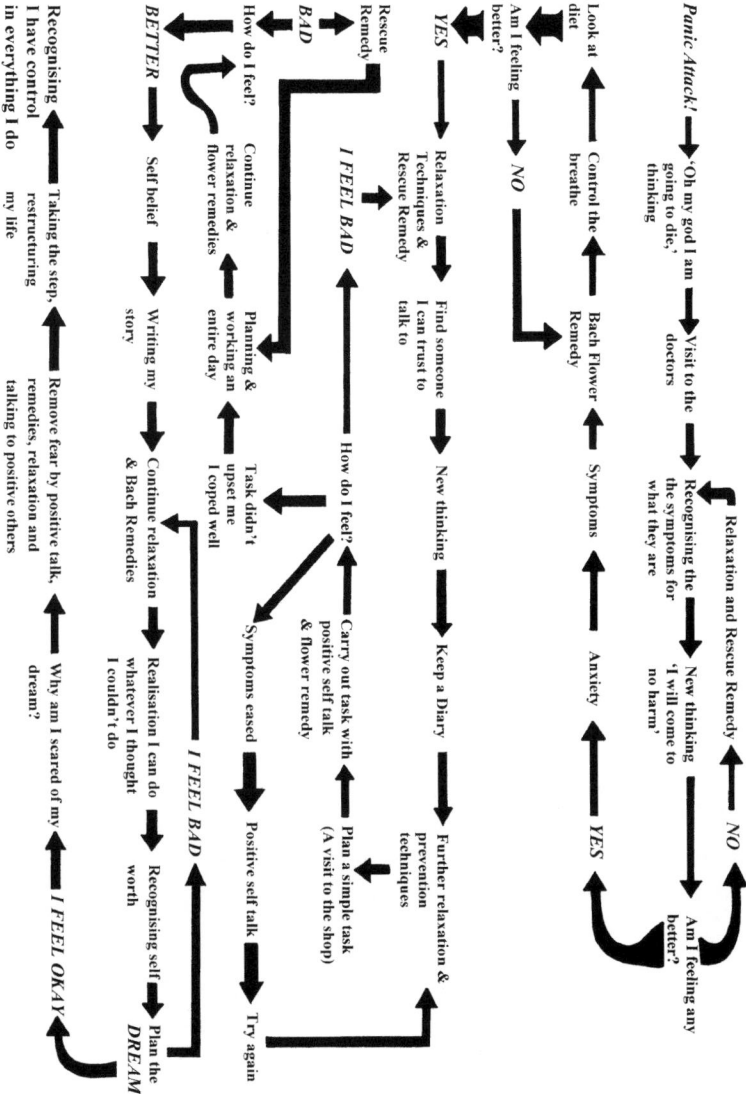

Panic Attack! → 'Oh my god I am going to die,' thinking → Visit to the doctors → Recognising the symptoms for what they are → New thinking 'I will come to no harm' → **NO** → Am I feeling any better?

Look at diet → Control the breathe → Bach Flower Remedy → Symptoms → Anxiety → **YES**

Am I feeling better? → **NO**

YES → Relaxation Techniques & Rescue Remedy → Find someone I can trust to talk to → New thinking → Keep a Diary → Further relaxation & prevention techniques

BAD → Rescue Remedy

Rescue Remedy → **I FEEL BAD** → How do I feel? → Carry out task with positive self talk & flower remedy → Plan a simple task (A visit to the shop)

How do I feel? → Continue relaxation & flower remedies → Planning & working an entire day → Task didn't upset me I coped well → Symptoms eased → Positive self talk → Try again

BETTER → Self belief → Writing my story → Continue relaxation & Bach Remedies → Realisation I can do whatever I thought I couldn't do → Recognising self worth → Plan the **DREAM**

I FEEL BAD

Recognising I have control in everything I do → Taking the step, restructuring my life → Remove fear by positive talk, remedies, relaxation and talking to positive others → Why am I scared of my dream? → **I FEEL OKAY**

Relaxation and Rescue Remedy → **NO** → Am I feeling any better?

New thinking → **YES**

295

- 26 -

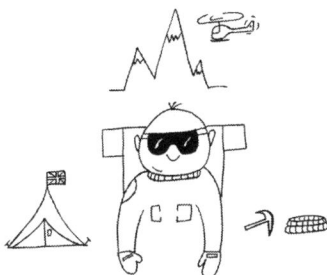

Survival Kit

When a panic attack strikes it can be difficult to know what to do, which is why I've compiled the most worthwhile techniques into one easy to read format. The survival kit is designed to ease the symptoms and help you between attacks when you feel under the weather.

The immediate attack!

I want you to control your breathing, it's become fast and shallow so we need to calm everything down.

Exercise 1 – Slowing down your breathing

Firstly, don't force the breath, try and keep it at an even speed. Preferably with a small pause in between. This method of controlled breathing removes all tingling sensations and pains in the chest, bringing you gently back to normal.

Keep the thoughts primarily on the breathing and not what's happening elsewhere, which will help calm the symptoms.

Take Rescue Remedy every few minutes

Tip: *'If you happen to have a paper bag lying around, like a popcorn bag, inhale and exhale into it. This recycles the carbon dioxide diminishing the panicky feelings. Otherwise, hold your breath for 10 seconds and then continue controlled breathing. - Repeat this as necessary.'*

Mental approach

Don't breed more fear by fearing what is happening with your body and mind. Allow the feelings to wash over you without the panicky thinking there is something wrong with you. There is nothing wrong with you, your body is just having an anxiety attack. *'THIS WILL PASS.'*

Talk with someone understanding

Talk with somebody you feel safe with and rationalise the panic along with the symptoms. This is a great way to dispel the anxiety.

Distract

Distraction like a good movie is helpful through difficult times. Sip your Rescue Remedy and lie down on the sofa with a blanket and rest. Keep telling yourself you are okay.

Meditate

Meditate the moment you feel you can achieve this without feeling too uncomfortable, and most importantly concentrate fully. Meditation will bring you back to a state of calm.

Relax

Relax and not feel guilty for doing so. Don't allow your mind to worry that you haven't done the dishes, or the hoovering, or called into the shops for some shopping. It doesn't matter right now. Time Out.

Sleep

Get some sleep. Time and sleep are the best healers for helping with anxiety.

Breathing exercise 2

Tools: You will need three books (not too heavy)

Find somewhere comfortable, but reasonably firm to lay down. Now place the books over the spot where your belly button is. What we're going to do is strengthen your breathing apparatus. The books are acting like weights in the gym and a good visual aid making sure the breath is coming from low down.

By doing this regularly, starting with five minutes a day slowly extending a further minute a week, your breathing will transfer from upper chest to lower chest, where it's supposed to be.

The task

I want you to exhale through your mouth, making sure all air is squeezed out. Good. Now breathe in through your mouth from deep down in your tummy, and hold. - Count to five, and release through mouth to the count of six. When you feel comfortable with this, try counting to six on the intake, and release to seven. And again, count to seven, release to eight. Eight to nine. And finally nine to nine. Every time you do this, notice how the books rise and fall, and try and keep their movement constant. Work with

---

this method and your breathing apparatus will strengthen, giving you better control over the attacks themselves.

Tip: *'For extra benefit, find a place with clean air for this exercise, such as a beach or hillside where the air is charged with beneficial ions.'*

Warding off the attack

You'll soon recognise the onset of a coming attack. This might start with a detachment from your surroundings. Maybe a deep fear death is near, sickness to the stomach, shaking, tightening of the chest and neck muscles, a sudden shortness of breath.

When this happens, do the following exercise.

Stand or sit away from whatever you are doing for a few minutes to gain control. You need to slow down your breathing to bring calm. Do this firstly by squeezing out all the air from your lungs through your mouth. Clear your mind and take a full in-breath through the mouth. Hold for three, exhale to the count of three.

Breathe in, hold for four, exhale to the count of four.

Continue to a max of nine until feelings subside.

Use 'Rescue Remedy' regularly.

You may find once you stop doing the exercise, panic returns minutes later. In this case, repeat the exercise again. Your subconscious will recognise you're serious here and calm is wanted, not a needless fight or flight response.

'Keeping your body in a state of calm breaks the pattern of panic attacks, eventually eliminating the trigger that has become so sensitive.'

Jin Shin Jyutsu

Jin Shin is an ancient healing art which can be extremely beneficial for the panic attack sufferer. It involves gently pressing on the skin releasing blocked energy around the body.

Typically, a session with a healer will last one hour, but I have included a few exercises to start you on your way.

What should you get from Jin Shin

A feeling of inner calm. It gives a sense of wholeness, relieving whatever physical and emotional problems you are dealing with at the moment.

We are after all energy beings, and when that energy becomes blocked or choked, we become ill. Free the energy flow and we resume good health.

The translation for Jin Shin Jyutsu is, 'art of the creator through compassionate and knowing man.'

Note: *'A sure sign this is working is stomach gurgling, followed by tension release in the muscles. But remember to drink plenty of water afterwards and then get plenty of rest.'*

'A good time to do the following exercises is just before bedtime. Jin Shin starts the healing process and can make you feel quite tired, sleep is an excellent remedy towards self healing.'

Exercise One – Calming the self

Lie down. Allow half an hour to do all three if you can, but any time is better than nothing.

Place back of right hand under body lying next to opposite hip.

Place left hand on opposite inner thigh where comfortable. Hold gently, no pressing. Keep position until a pulse can be felt in both hands, this indicates the flow of energy.

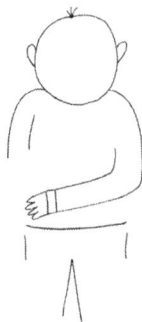

Right hand on opposite hip, left on opposite inner thigh.

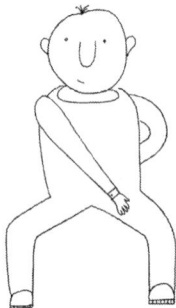

Left hand on opposite hip, right on opposite inner thigh.

Note. *'It might take several sessions until a pulse may be felt, so as a guide, do this for five minutes at a time.'*

Now take left hand from inner thigh, place on side of neck with fingers wide spread covering area from back of ear to shoulder. Hold.

Now repeat entire exercise but the other way round. Left hand under body next to opposite hip, right hand on opposite inner thigh etc.

Exercise Two – Taking tension out from upper chest

A distressing symptom like tension in the chest can be relieved with this very simple technique. Concentrate on the breath while doing this and try and not let your panicky thoughts run away with you. You can beat anxiety; you are doing remarkably well.

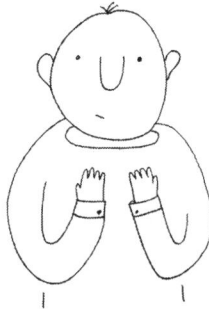

Hold fingers either side of breast bone three ribs down from collar bone. Hold, breathe, and imagine a white light filling your body. - **Say, *'I am safe.'***

Do this as many times during the day as you like, and as long as you like, to find relief.

Exercise three -Hand work

Note. *'This is very easy to do. You can do these when chatting to somebody or watching T.V.'*

Index finger – Kidneys (release fear). Hold with other hand. Circle ring finger. Helps Breathing by opening up lungs. If time, hold each finger in turn.

(See picture below).

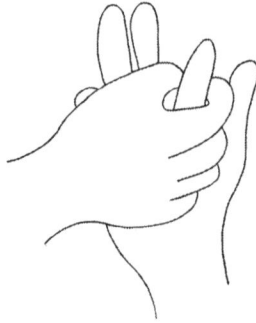

That should get you started and feeling more human. Repeat daily, and don't forget to look up someone who does Jin Shin, as their time spent on you will be invaluable.

Moving from the dark into the light

A visualization technique this one. Negative patterns bring darkness. But as light brings comfort and healing, it makes sense to move into the light. We can do this as many times as we like by visualising the following.

'Find a quiet moment and get comfortable. Close your eyes and imagine a shaft of white light emitting from the sky. See how bright and wondrous the light is and feel the energy it projects. Now walk forward towards the light, stand in the centre and see the light all around you. It's so bright, but it doesn't harm your eyes. Stand there for a few minutes absorbing the power it gives.'

Grounding

Grounding is very important if you want to keep your feet securely on the ground. Otherwise you feel light headed, and it becomes extremely difficult to take in what's happening around you. When we're in this state, we feel anxious, and are more easily influenced by the thoughts and emotions of others.

Grounding is vital for panic attack sufferers

Simple grounding techniques.

1. *'Stand in your garden or a nearby park with your shoes and socks off. Close your eyes and imagine roots growing from your feet tunnelling deep into the earth.'*

2. *'See yourself out of focus, then slowly bring yourself back into focus.'*

3. *'Stamp your feet and pat your body all over.'*

Protective bubble

Protective bubble's strength lies in stopping negative energies from attacking us. Think of it like, a giant, all enveloping see through shield, keeping you from harm in moments of crisis. Or as a protector, while you're in busy spaces where everybody's energies can leave you tired and depleted.

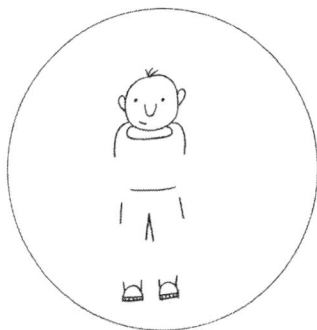

'Imagine you are surrounded by a see through membrane, a protective skin. Stand or sit a moment just feeling the energy around you. Breathe deeply.'

Say to yourself: *'Only good energy can penetrate my bubble, negative energy will bounce clean off.'* Get used to *the bubble itself, then finally exhale slowly and open your eyes feeling relaxed and protected.'*

Protective bubble can be done wherever you are, and has the added advantage of only taking a few moments. – Try and do this once in the morning, and again before bedtime.

Cleansing shower

When taking a shower, just imagine the water removing all the stresses and strains from your body. See the colour of the stress as it hits the shower tray and runs down the plug hole. Keep this up until the water in your mind runs clear.

Purple light

Purple is one of the colours of healing. Imagine you are standing within a column of beautiful purple light, and relax in the knowledge you are safe.

Dispelling negativity

Instead of saying, 'I hate this lousy weather', say, *'I love the weather today.'* Instead of saying, 'I hate this traffic jam', say, *'I love these moments because I have time to think.'*

Every time something comes up during the day you hate, protest about, or just plainly can't stand, turn it around in your head to a positive. If you feel rough, say, *'I am getting stronger.'*

Other tips

Wear a Q-Link

A health pendant that reduces stress and enhances your energy. I personally wear one and find it very beneficial. - Available from many online stores or auction sites.

Bach flower remedy

When you're feeling rotten, don't forget to increase your dosage. A couple of drops every ten minutes will steadily bring you back.

'Remember to take remedies even when you feel okay. This will help prevent future panic attacks from occurring.'

Bach remedy bath

Take a relaxing bath and add Rescue Remedy with Rock Water. This enhances the calming effect.

Incense sticks

Incense sticks can enhance relaxation, great to light just before meditating.

Be healed

Have a healer work on you regularly. Also seek out some healing fairs, where you'll meet some interesting people who will be only too glad to help.

EFT

Use some emotional freedom techniques. A highly effective self help therapy that can diminish what you are feeling right now. Simple and easy too! (Books available online).

Counselling

Find a trusted someone you can talk to. Don't be afraid of telling them what you are feeling and the thoughts currently going around your mind. Unloading will calm the anxiety.

Look after yourself

Don't push yourself. It's time to relax and just chill, calming all your body's systems down instead of all that rush.

No pressure

Don't pressure yourself into doing something you feel you can't do. Say *'NO'* without feeling guilty. You need to look after yourself and get better.

Clearing the mind

Try to stop your mind racing with energy wasting thoughts, they heighten tension and bring in panic and thoughts of, *'I'm losing control.'*

Sit somewhere peaceful and relax every muscle in your body. Breathe deeply. Now close your eyes and I want you to imagine there is a wooden box in front of you. Take your problems as they pop into your head and place them in the box. Do this regularly to feel calmness with clarity.

Spider hands

This is a simple way of unblocking energy throughout the entire body. A good point to note is, if the mind is full, you can unblock with the spider hand technique.

Symptoms such as heavy head, panicky feelings, pains that come and go, all point to energy which is not flowing as it should. The beauty with this technique is you can literally do it anywhere and nobody will be the wiser.

Use spider hands as often as you can. Just sit quietly, hold the fingertips gently together, and regulate your breathing like I have shown you.

You can even try adding some visualization such as a healing shaft of purple or white light. - Bask in the radiance, trust the feelings will pass soon. (Practice regularly and you'll improve).

'YOU ARE SAFE'

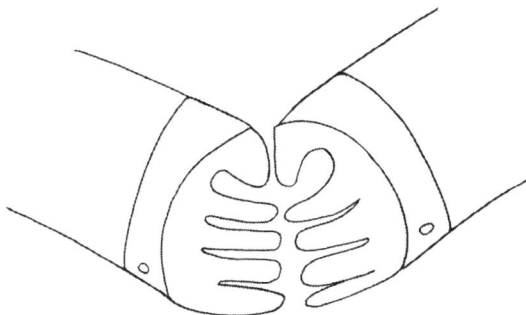

Spider hands

Posture

While we're on the subject of energy flow, posture is worthy of a mention here. Think of a kinked hose when we hunch over and grip our muscles tight, because it's the only way we can stand the pain. The flow is disrupted, creating pain. Stand tall and allow the energy to flow freely.

It may feel uncomfortable at first but it makes a big difference.

Make a list

To control uncontrollable mind panic, or what I like to call headless chicken syndrome, make a list of all the jobs you have to do. This will stop your mind racing from one job to the next without actually achieving any of them. Tick when done and don't forget to congratulate yourself.

Clearing the mind

Write destructive thoughts on a piece of paper and tear them up proving they have no place with you. This will bring calmness of mind. Don't' forget to replace them with positives and remind yourself of these positives on a regular basis.

(Take Rescue Remedy)

Believe

Believe in the methods you try from this book. Belief holds immense power, sustaining the route towards your success. Remember, *you can do it!*

Summary

Tick

Box

☐Breathing correctly keeps the entire body system calm.

☐When an attack threatens, step back a moment and do the breathing exercise until it passes.

☐Don't feed more fear into the anxiety. Allow the sensations to pass by.

☐Use distraction to remove emphasis from what's happening inside.

☐Jin Shin techniques can be used as often as you like.

☐Time to move from the dark into the light.

☐Grounding brings back a connection with reality.

☐Protective bubble stops people's emotions attacking or draining you.

☐Turn negative thoughts into positive ones.

☐Keep a bottle of Bach flower 'Rescue Remedy' at hand. Take drops at the slightest hint of an attack or whenever you feel anxious.

☐Take remedies throughout the day to help prevent future panic attacks and anxiety.

☐Try EFT (Emotional Freedom Technique).

☐Meditate.

☐Follow the techniques in this book and you will make strides towards better health and eventually beating this disorder.

☐Read chapter 17 on coping strategies.

☐Don't give up.

☐You are way stronger than you believe you are.

☐Remember, 'YOU ARE SAFE.'

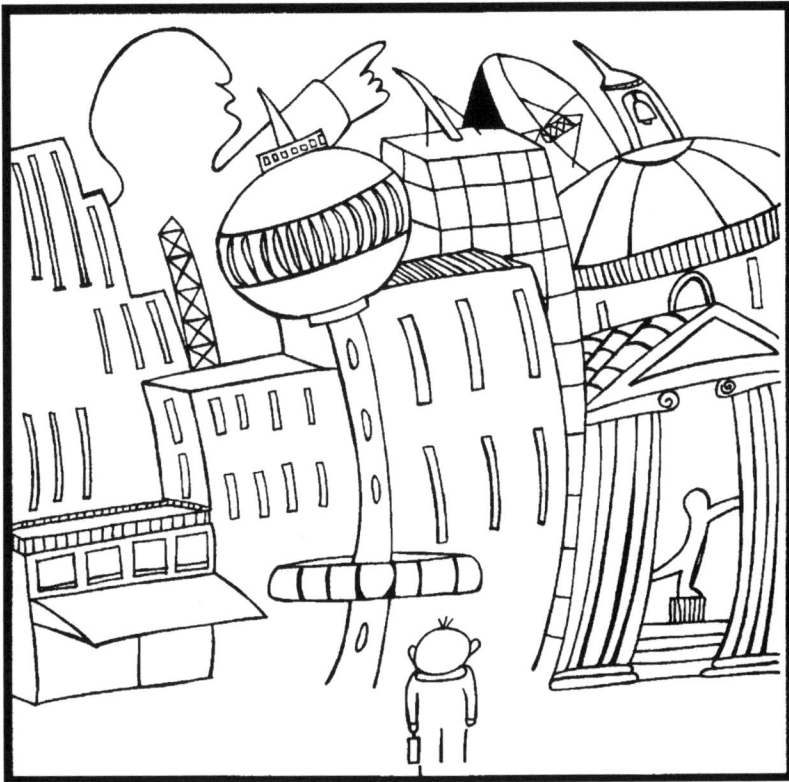

- 27 -

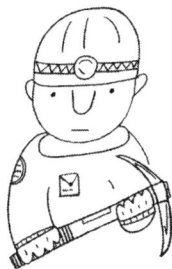

Back in Control – Q&A

Today seems a different world away from those years I suffered from panic. Those were difficult times, but now I can say hand on heart for the majority the attacks have subsided. Flare-ups can happen from time to time, but that's just an indicator I need to readdress something in my life and things will return to normality once more.

You will come to recognise this in your own life as well.

It is quite natural to fall back into your old patterns, but learning to recognise how these patterns are detrimental to your well being is half of the battle.

To give you an example, recently I had a lot of work on and this was draining me physically, but it wasn't until I started to have sleepless nights that I realised I had fallen back into one of my old patterns of pushing myself too hard. This resulted in feelings of anxiousness and pains in the chest.

By writing down how I felt it became all too obvious where I needed to make changes again.

I realised:

O I had been pushing myself too hard.

O I hadn't been taking time out to rest.

O I'd been eating irregularly or the wrong type of foods.

O I hadn't been concentrating on my breathing.

O I'd forgotten to take my remedies.

O I had relaxed on my meditation routine.

O I'd been allowing negative thinking to get a hold of me.

And that's just how easy it can be done. Just by sitting down with a pen and a piece of paper, five minutes later I knew how to change my life so well being would return.

I encourage you to do the same. Whenever the feeling of anxiousness encompasses you, sit down and write what you have been doing for the past few days. And if you can't see it, pass it over to somebody else, because quite often we can't see the problem yet a fresh set of eyes can.

Things to check to see if you are over doing things:

Bedtime – Are you getting enough quality sleep, or are you staying up to watch the late movie?

Food – Are you eating the right foods and at the right times? If we miss food this stresses the system. Incorrect food can heighten anxiety e.g. sweets.

Work – Are you still thinking about work after clocking off? Have you signed up for too much overtime?

Chill out time – Have you had many moments where you just sit and relax, or are you just rushing around all the time?

Now it's easier to see the changes you need to make. It might be you get home late and go to bed with your head spinning. You just need to switch off and get some relaxation time in before bedtime. That could be it. Balance resumed.

It's very easy to fall off the log, so to speak, but it's counterproductive to become angry and discouraged. This only stalls your healing. Far better to identify what's needed and go from there.

Q&A - Common questions:

Can panic be controlled successfully?

Yes. I don't suffer full blown panic attacks anymore, and I have learnt to deal with the minor ones. Be patient with yourself and persistence really pays off.

When will this ever stop?

I can't say when, everybody is different, but you will start to feel better over the coming weeks.

Why has this happened to me?

By working through the exercises you'll come to understand why, and how to overcome panic and anxiety.

Will things settle down and will I feel normal again?

Yes. By re-teaching your body and mind how to relax, and not to expect panic, things will return to a normal state.

Will I have flare ups?

It can happen, but you will get better at preventing them. You'll learn by keeping an eye on the way you control stress in your life, and the way you treat your body, flare ups will be few and far between.

Why flower remedies?

Helps you feel emotionally stronger while putting things back in perspective. This gives you the confidence, strength and support to move forward.

Can I overdose on the flower remedies?

No. They are 100% safe. They can be taken alongside any medication you are on. But if you are concerned, consult your doctor first.

What if I take remedies that I don't need?

The body will absorb the remedies it needs and ignore the ones it doesn't.

Why use Rescue Remedy?

Rescue Remedy brings everything back into perspective and calms the panics/anxiety.

Where can I buy Rescue Remedy?

Chemists, supermarkets and online stores.

Visit: www.creaturecomforters.co.uk

Where do I find a practitioner?

Try via the web, complimentary therapy centres or healing fairs.

How does energy healing work?

The healer raises his energy and offers it to you. And because your energy is in a low state (unwell), it lifts you and brings your levels to the same energy of your healer. When this happens, the body is able to repair itself. Combine with flower remedies, and you'll find the treatment of anxiety can be very effective.

Can I have too much healing?

No. The body will only accept what it needs.

Will complimentary therapy help, why not take regular medicine?

Both complement each other. Therapies harmonise the body and mind bringing it back into a balanced state. Where medicine, (beta blockers) work, by blocking the messages that cause the symptoms of the fight & flight response.

I'm on medication already, can I still use therapies?

Yes. But if you're still worried, consult your doctor beforehand.

What if I don't believe in complimentary therapies?

Flower remedies and healing can work whether or not the patient believes in it. But I urge you to go open minded on this one, because quite often belief speeds and enhances the healing process.

I find it difficult to visualise

Try using a CD or tape. Just the intent of seeing a white light has the same benefits as seeing it in your head. Concentrate on the feelings in your body it brings. – **Note. Don't try too hard. Relax, let the image be formed naturally.**

Why do we use white light in meditations?

White light holds all the colours we are made of. By using white light, we feel the maximum benefits without having to go through each colour in turn.

Why do I feel fine until I go into a particular situation?

If you panic, say in a crowd, you will likely panic when you revisit the situation. Controlled exposure (See, *'To walk the Devils Yard'*) will deal with this. Also try hypnotherapy and EFT therapy.

Why do some people make me feel uncomfortable?

For the moment this is something you will have to just accept. Don't put any necessary pressure on yourself by being around these kind of people. Stay around those who you feel safe and comfortable with.

Is there anything I can wear that will make me feel better and less stressful?

Try a Q-Link. The Q-Link reduces stress and anxiety while raising your energy levels.

My mind is on overdrive

Try taking *'White Chestnut'* and *'Vervain'* Bach flower remedies. Write your thoughts on paper.

Why do I jump at every little thing?

You have to remember your senses are set to a heightened level of alert right now (Fight or Flight). These will diminish as you progress.

I feel I can't relax, I feel I must keep moving all the time

The adrenaline makes you want to keep going, and the body is responding to this. You need to re-teach your body relaxation and these feelings will subside. Healing, meditation, flower remedies are very good for this.

Why do I feel sick all the time?

The increase in adrenaline makes the stomach acid become more volatile. The reason being, our fight or flight response mode wants the stomach to be clear of food (by being sick) to get rid of excess weight. Less weight means you can run faster from a dangerous situation.

Why do I shake?

Excess of adrenaline and muscle tension.

The pains in my chest hurt. Am I having a heart attack?

Concerning panic attacks, sharp pains in the chest do not signify a heart attack. But if you are concerned, see a doctor. When you get the all clear, remember healing and flower remedies will be of help here. **Remember, if you are concerned, check with your doctor.**

The fear I feel seems so real

And it is. The body believes it's running from an extreme danger, but you will de-sensitize and these feelings will disappear.

I feel as though I'm going to die

Remember – this is a natural response (fight or flight) built into everyone of us on this planet. You are safe, you will get through this. - *Anxiety makes you feel this way.*

Will the pains in my body eventually go?

Yes they will. As the anxiety diminishes so will the pains.

I feel confused, I can't see a way out of this

Follow this book and you will come to understand yourself and how to be panic free for the rest of your life.

Am I crazy?

Most definitely not. Don't think this or allow others to impose this kind of thinking upon you. You are working through a life changing experience right now, you will emerge far stronger.

I hate myself

The panic and feelings of fear become too much which can lead to this type of thinking. Write down the positives about yourself and take the following flower remedies. – *'Rock Water,'* *'Holly,' and 'Crab Apple.'*

Is it normal to have such feelings of extreme anger?

Repressed emotions rewrite our thinking which can lead to extremes of anger. But you will learn to release the anger and negative feelings you have for others and situations, and these feelings will dissolve.

Does my state of mind have anything to do with panic and anxiety, and the pains in my body?

Yes. Once you have learnt to release the triggers that cause the panic, the body will not enter the fight or flight response. The pains will then go.

I feel so tired and drained, how can I possibly do any of what you have described?

In this situation, try Bach flower remedies, healing by a practitioner along with plenty of rest. When your energies raise a little, you will be able to continue with the rest of the healing process.

I can't stand this anymore!!!

I myself was at this stage of thinking. But just hold in there, because with the flower remedies, healing and changing your mind set, things will get easier faster than you may think.

'Don't give up on yourself. You will get through this.'

And don't be afraid to ask for help. Find a practitioner that can assist you through this period of your life. Do not see this as a weakness.

Can I return to the exercises in the book whenever I want?

Yes. In fact I encourage you to do so. Keeping on top of things will keep the panics away.

Summary

Tick

Box

☐Don't beat yourself up. Anger will only fan the flames.

☐Take time out, relax.

☐Eat good food.

☐Take multivitamins. (Unless you can't for health issues).

☐Meditate.

☐Find yourself a practitioner and have some healing.

☐Take your flower remedies every ten minutes. (If you only have 'Rescue Remedy,' take that).

☐Write down what has happened over the past few days and see where you can change things for the better.

☐Remove stressful situations, or if that's not possible, try and not let things get to you. Write the things that bother you down to get them out of your head.

☐It's okay to say '**NO**' to people and situations. Honour yourself.

☐Try wearing a Q-Link.

☐Health and being supported are the most important things. Anything else is just costume jewellery.

☐Panic is not a bad thing. It's just our body warning us we need to look after ourselves a bit better.

☐If you feel you need to, repeat the exercises in this book. Remember, you are just recognising where you need to make changes.

☐'YOU ARE SAFE.'

About the Author

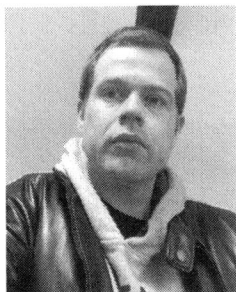

Richard Hathaway lives in Norfolk England and has suffered panic attacks in his past. He always vowed that when he made the often difficult journey back from this disorder, he would write about it, and help others who found themselves in the same situation.

Through grit and determination, and a burning desire to get the answers, he has put his voice on paper for others to follow and find relief from what can be a harrowing experience.

It's fair to say, Panic Attacks are a subject close to his heart, but Richard also has an interest in fiction, and aims to publish a novel in the not too distant future.

You can visit his website at: www.astara-publications.com

Also try:

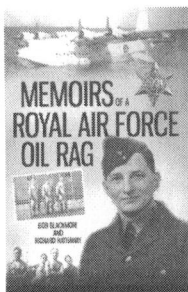

Memoirs of a Royal Air Force Oil Rag

By Bob Blackmore & Richard Hathaway

Available in hardback, paperback, and

ebook formats.

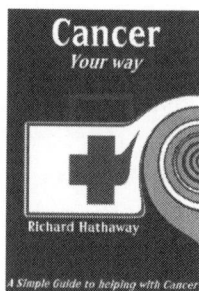

Cancer Your Way
By Richard Hathaway
Available in paperback and
ebook formats.

Thank you for Reading

'I would be very grateful if you would leave a review of this publication on the outlet you purchased from. Thank you.'

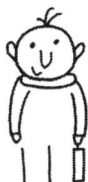

7140583R00182

Printed in Great Britain
by Amazon.co.uk, Ltd.,
Marston Gate.